COUNTER

for Branded Foods

COLLINS GEM

CALORIE COUNTER

for Branded Foods

COLLINS
London and Glasgow

First published 1984
Reprint 10 9 8 7 6

© William Collins Sons and Company Limited 1984

ISBN 0 00 458762 6
Printed in Great Britain

CONTENTS

INTRODUCTION

Diets come and diets go, but still the most reliable way of losing weight – or of maintaining a sensible weight – is by counting Calories.

The energy the body needs to survive is generated from the nutrients – carbohydrates, fats, proteins and vitamins – in the food we eat. When we consume in this form more energy than our bodies use up in our daily life, then we put on weight. About half the energy used up by the body in a day is needed to enable it just to survive – this is the basic metabolism rate – while the other half is taken up by activity, by work or play. Generally speaking, people who do more need more and can consume more. A miner expends more energy than an office worker, a docker more than a driver, a squash player more than a golfer. In the following pages there are tables which give the average energy used in a day doing certain jobs, and the energy used in an hour taking part in certain activities. But, for reasons still not perfectly understood by scientists, not everyone uses up the same amount of energy doing the same job or playing the same game; we each have to determine our own energy needs and decide for ourselves how much food energy we need to consume.

Also included among the tables are those for desirable weights according to height and frame. It has been calculated that one pound of body fat is equal to 3500 Calories, so for every pound required to be lost, 3500 Calories must come out of the diet – but not all at once! Anyone considering trying to lose a lot of weight should consult their doctor, and those just keen not to overdo it should remember that the best way to lose weight – or not to put it on – is to eat a sensible diet and to eat in moderation.

The most convenient form of measurement of the energy value of food for non-scientific use is the kilocalorie, or Calorie, which is what is given here. The foods are listed in **bold roman type** in alphabetical order in the left-hand column of each page; the name of the manufacturer is in the second column; and the energy values are given per 100 grams (3.5 ounces) in the third column. Where at all possible and available, in the last column Calorie values per portion or pack are given. If such information is not available, then the Calorie value per ounce has been given. Unbranded foods and Calorie values listed in ***bold italic type*** have been obtained with permission from *The Composition of Foods,* published by Her Majesty's Stationery Office.

The publishers are grateful to all the manufacturers who gave information on their products. The list of foods included is as up to date as it was possible to make it, but it should be remembered that new food products are frequently put on the market and existing ones withdrawn, so it has not been possible to include everything. If you cannot find a particular food here, you can still, however, obtain a guideline figure by finding an equivalent product from a different manufacturer.

Weights and measures

Imperial to Metric

1 ounce (oz) = 28.35 grams (g)
1 pound (lb) = 453.60 grams (g)
1 fluid ounce (fl. oz) = 29.57 millilitres (ml)
1 pint = 0.568 litre

Metric to Imperial

100 grams (g) = 3.53 ounces (oz)
1 kilogram (kg) = 2.2 pounds (lb)
100 millilitres (ml) = 3.38 fluid ounces (fl. oz)
1 litre = 1.76 pints

Abbreviations

These have been avoided wherever possible, but of necessity some have had to be used. They are:

BHS: British Home Stores	oz: ounces
fl. oz: fluid ounces	sm: small
g: grams	st: stone/s
in: inch/inches	std: standard
inc: including	straw: strawberry
kgs: kilograms	svg: serving
lb: pound/s	tbs: tablespoon
m: metre/s	tbsp: tablespoon
med: medium	van: vanilla
ml: millilitres	veg: vegetable/s
negl: negligible	

Average daily Calorie expenditure, by occupation

Men		Women	
Sedentary			
Retired	2300	Elderly	
Office workers	2500	housewives	1980
Lab technicians	2850	Middle-aged	
Drivers, pilots,		housewives	2075
teachers, journalists,			
professional people,			
shop workers	2700		
Building workers	3000		
Moderately active			
University students	2950	Lab technicians	2125
Light industry,		Shop workers	2250
railway workers,		Univ. students	2300
postmen, joiners,		Factory workers	2320
farm workers	3000	Office workers	2200
Very active			
Steel workers	3250	Bakery workers, some	
Some farm workers	3450	factory workers	2500
Army cadets and			
recruits	3500		
Miners, forestry			
workers, dockers, some			
building workers	3600		

Average hourly Calorie requirement, by activity:

	Women	Men
Bowling	207	270
Cycling: moderate	192	256
hard	507	660
Dancing: ballroom	264	352
Domestic work	153	200
Driving	108	144
Eating	84	112
Gardening: active	276	368
Golf	144	192
Ironing	120	160
Office work: active	120	160
Rowing	600	800
Running: moderate	444	592
hard	692	900
Sewing and knitting	84	112
Sitting at rest	84	112
Skiing	461	600
Squash	461	600
Swimming: moderate	230	300
hard	480	640
Table tennis	300	400
Tennis	336	448
Typing	108	144
Walking: moderate	168	224

Desirable weights of adults

Small frame: men and women
Height without shoes

Men

ft in	m	st lb	st lb	kgs
4 8	1.42			
4 9	1.45			
4 10	1.47			
4 11	1.50			
5 0	1.52			
5 1	1.55	8 0–	8 8	50.8–54.4
5 2	1.58	8 3–	8 12	52.2–56.3
5 3	1.60	8 6–	9 0	53.5–57.2
5 4	1.63	8 9–	9 3	54.9–58.5
5 5	1.65	8 12–	9 7	56.3–60.3
5 6	1.68	9 2–	9 11	58.1–62.1
5 7	1.70	9 6–	10 1	59.9–64
5 8	1.73	9 10–	10 5	61.7–65.8
5 9	1.75	10 0–	10 10	63.5–68
5 10	1.78	10 4–	11 0	65.3–69.9
5 11	1.80	10 8–	11 4	67.1–71.7
6 0	1.83	10 12–	11 8	69 –73.5
6 1	1.85	11 2–	11 13	70.8–75.8
6 2	1.88	11 6–	12 3	72.6–77.6
6 3	1.91	11 10–	12 7	74.4–79.4

Women

st lb	st lb	kgs
6 8–	7 0	41.7–44.5
6 10–	7 3	42.6–45.8
6 12–	7 6	43.6–47.2
7 1–	7 9	44.9–48.5
7 4–	7 12	46.3–49.9
7 7–	8 1	47.6–51.3
7 10–	8 4	49 –52.6
7 13–	8 7	50.4–54
8 2–	8 11	51.7–55.8
8 6–	9 1	53.5–57.6
8 10–	9 5	55.3–59.4
9 0–	9 9	57.2–61.2
9 4–10	0	59 –63.5
9 8–10	4	60.8–65.3
9 12–10	8	62.6–67.1

Desirable weights of adults

Medium frame: men and women
Height without shoes

Men

ft in	m	st lb	st lb	kgs
4 8	1.42			
4 9	1.45			
4 10	1.47			
4 11	1.50			
5 0	1.52			
5 1	1.55	8 6-	9 3	53.5-58.5
5 2	1.58	8 9-	9 7	54.9-60.3
5 3	1.60	8 12-	9 10	56.3-61.7
5 4	1.63	9 1-	9 13	57.6-63.1
5 5	1.65	9 4-	10 3	59 -64.9
5 6	1.68	9 8-	10 7	60.8-66.8
5 7	1.70	9 12-	10 12	62.6-69
5 8	1.73	10 2-	11 2	64.4-70.8
5 9	1.75	10 6-	11 6	66.2-72.6
5 10	1.78	10 10-	11 11	68 -74.8
5 11	1.80	11 0-	12 1	69.9-77.1
6 0	1.83	11 4-	12 7	71.7-79.4
6 1	1.85	11 8-	12 12	73.5-81.7
6 2	1.88	11 13-	13 3	75.8-83.9
6 3	1.91	12 4-	13 8	78 -86.2

Women

st lb	st lb	kgs
6 12-	7 9	43.6-48.5
7 0-	7 12	44.5-49.9
7 3-	8 1	45.8-51.3
7 6-	8 4	47.2-52.6
7 9-	8 7	48.5-54
7 12-	8 10	49.9-55.3
8 1-	9 0	51.3-57.2
8 4-	9 4	52.6-59
8 8-	9 9	54.4-61.2
8 12-	9 13	56.3-63.1
9 2-	10 3	58.1-64.9
9 6-	10 7	59.9-66.7
9 10-	10 11	61.7-68.5
10 0-	11 1	63.5-70.3
10 4-	11 5	65.3-72.1

Desirable weights of adults

Large frame: men and women
Height without shoes

			Men			Women		
ft	in	m	st lb	st lb	kgs	st lb	st lb	kgs
4	8	1.42				7 6–	8 7	47.2–54
4	9	1.45				7 8–	8 10	48.1–55.3
4	10	1.47				7 11–	8 13	49.4–56.7
4	11	1.50				8 0–	9 2	50.8–58.1
5	0	1.52				8 3–	9 5	52.2–59.4
5	1	1.55	9 0–10	1	57.2–64	8 6–	9 8	53.5–60.8
5	2	1.58	9 3–10	4	58.5–65.3	8 9–	9 12	54.9–62.6
5	3	1.60	9 6–10	8	59.9–67.1	8 13–	10 2	56.7–64.4
5	4	1.63	9 9–10	12	61.2–69	9 3–10	6	58.5–66.2
5	5	1.65	9 12–11	2	62.6–70.8	9 7–10	10	60.3–68
5	6	1.68	10 2–11	7	64.4–73	9 11–11	0	62.1–69.9
5	7	1.70	10 7–11	12	66.7–75.3	10 1–11	4	64 –71.7
5	8	1.73	10 11–12	2	68.5–77.1	10 5–11	9	65.8–73.9
5	9	1.75	11 1–12	6	70.3–78.9	10 9–12	0	67.6–76.2
5	10	1.78	11 5–12	11	72.1–81.2	10 13–12	5	69.4–78.5
5	11	1.80	11 10–13	2	74.4–83.5			
6	0	1.83	12 0–13	7	76.2–85.7			
6	1	1.85	12 5–13	12	78.5–88			
6	2	1.88	12 10–14	3	80.7–90.3			
6	3	1.91	13 0–14	8	82.6–92.5			

Daily Calories for maintenance of desirable weight

Calculated for a moderately active life. If you are very active add 50 Calories; if your life is sedentary take away 75 Calories.

Weight		Age 18–35		Age 35–55		Age 55–75	
st lb	kgs	Men	Women	Men	Women	Men	Women
7 1	44.9		1700		1500		1300
7 12	49.9	2200	1850	1950	1650	1650	1400
8 9	54.9	2400	2000	2150	1750	1850	1550
9 2	58.1		2100		1900		1600
9 6	59.9	2550	2150	2300	1950	1950	1650
10 3	64.9	2700	2300	2400	2050	2050	1800
11 0	69.9	2900	2400	2600	2150	2200	1850
11 11	74.8	3100	2550	2800	2300	2400	1950
12 8	79.8	3250		2950		2500	
13 5	84.8	3300		3100		2600	

Product	Brand	Calories per 100g/ 100ml	Calories per oz/ pack/ portion
Abbey Crunch	McVitie		per biscuit 49
Aberdeen rolls	St Michael	421	119
Abernethy biscuits	Macfarlane Lang		per biscuit 66
Ackee, canned		*151*	*43*
Advocaat		*272*	*77*
Aero:	Rowntree		medium 210
milk chocolate	Mackintosh	525	large 435
orange		530	medium 205
peppermint		530	medium 205
After Eight mints	Rowntree Mackintosh	420	per mint 25
Albany Biscuits	Huntley & Palmers	497	per biscuit 39
Alfonal salad dressing	Alfonal	310	88
All butter biscuits	St Michael	481	per biscuit 46
All butter crunch biscuits	Sainsbury		per biscuit 30
All sauce	HP Foods	124	35
All-bran		*273*	*77*
All-Bran	Kellogg's	248	70
Allinson bread	St Michael	215	61
Almond biscuits	St Michael	522	per biscuit 49
Almond cake (round)	Tesco	420	119
Almond flakes	Sainsbury	582	165
	Tesco	582	165
	Whitworths	565	160
Almond iced tarts	Lyons	424	per tart 127
Almond layer cake	BHS	469	133

1

Product	Brand	Calories per 100g/ 100ml	Calories per oz/ pack/ portion
Almond slices	BHS	379	per slice 125
	Sainsbury		per slice 130
	Waitrose	395	112
Almonds,			
blanched	Tesco	582	165
dry roasted	Tesco	650	184
ground	Safeway	598	170
	Sainsbury	582	165
	Tesco	565	160
	Whitworths	565	160
sweet	Tesco	565	160
	Whitworths	555	157
whole		*565*	*160*
(with shells)		*210*	*60*
whole	Safeway	598	170
	Sainsbury	582	165
whole blanched	Whitworths	565	160
Alpen	Weetabix	375	1½oz (3 tbsp) 160 + 2oz milk 37 = 197
Alphabetti Spaghetti with tomato sauce	Crosse & Blackwell	61	17
Ambrosia products *see Rice, Sago, etc.*			
American ginger ale	Britvic	34	9.5
	Club	35	113ml 40 185ml 65
	Hunts	39	11
	Idris	28	8
	Safeway	20–30	6–9
	Schweppes	21	6
	Tesco	28	8

Product	Brand	Calories per 100g/ 100ml	Calories per oz/ pack/ portion
American ginger ale	Waitrose	28	8
low calorie	Club	negl.	negl.
	Hunts	1	
	Slimsta	4	1
	Tesco	6	2
slimline	Schweppes	0.35	
American dry ginger ale	Sainsbury	14	125ml/ ¼ pint 20
low calorie	Sainsbury	1.5	125ml/ ¼ pint 2
American salad	Eden Vale	141	40
Anchovy paste	Shippams	150	43
Angel cake	Sainsbury	405	¹/₅ cake/2oz 230
	Waitrose	525	122
Angel sandwich	BHS	448	per cake (250g) 1120
Angel sandwich cut cake	St Michael	574	163
Animal biscuits	Cadbury's	480	136
Apple *see also Bramley apple*			
Apple and blackberry crumble (baked)	Tiffany's	240	¼ crumble 270
Apple and blackberry jam	Tesco	279	79
Apple and blackberry pie filling	Pack-a-Pie	62	per pack 253
	Sainsbury	115	1tbsp/2oz 65
	Tesco	92	26
Apple and blackcurrant jam	Tesco	279	79

3

Product	Brand	Calories per 100g/ 100ml	Calories per oz/ pack/ portion
Apple and blackcurrant pie (dessert)	Harvest (Lyons)	316	per pie 1005
(individual)	Harvest (Lyons)	322	per pie 354
(small)	Lyons	356	per pie 176
Apple and blackcurrant puff pastries	Lyons	404	per pastry 186
Apple and damson jam	Tesco	279	79
Apple and date dessert bar	Prewetts	232	66
Apple and plum jam	Tesco	279	79
Apple and raspberry jam	Tesco	279	79
Apple and raspberry pie filling	Pack-a-Pie Tesco	63 66	per pack 256 19
Apple and strawberry jam	Tesco	279	79
Apple Barrel drink	Libby	40	11
Apple chutney		*193*	*55*
Apple cream dessert	St Michael	170	48
Apple crumble		*208*	*59*
Apple crumble, chunkey (baked)	Tiffany's	310	¼ crumble 350
Apple crush, sparkling	Waitrose	34	9.5
Apple juice	Sainsbury Tesco	46 45	¼ pint 65 13

4

Product	Brand	Calories per 100g/ 100ml	Calories per oz/ pack/ portion
Apple juice			
pure	Waitrose	37	11
UHT	BHS	45	13
Apple juice/apple juice drink	H.P. Bulmer	38	11
Apple juice drink	Shloer	35	10
Apple pie			
(4 portion)	Sainsbury		¼ pie 250
	St Michael	301	85
	Waitrose	190	54
(dessert)	Harvest (Lyons)	322	per pie 1024
(individual)	Harvest (Lyons)	323	per pie 355
(small)	Lyons	355	per pie 176
Apple pie filling	Pack-a-Pie	65	per pack 265
	Tesco	64	18
	Waitrose	95	27
Apple pies (6 per pack)	St Michael	323	per pie 192
Apple pudding (foil basin)	Sainsbury		whole 570
Apple puff pastries	Lyons	425	per pastry 196
Apple puffs	St Michael	376	per puff 200
Apple sauce	Colman's	80	23
	Heinz	65	18
Apple sauce mix (as sold)	Colman's	380	108
	Knorr	362	23g pack 83
Apple slices	John West	31	9
Dutch	St Michael	212	per cake 190

Product	Brand	Calories per 100g/ 100ml	Calories per oz/ pack/ portion
Apple sponge	St Michael	240	68
Apple tarts			
(2 per pack)	Sainsbury		per tart 250
(4 per pack)	St Michael	278	per tart 160
Apples, cooking			
baked (with skin)		31	9
baked without sugar		39	11
raw		37	10
stewed with sugar		66	19
stewed without sugar		32	9
Apples, eating		46	13
(with skin and core)		35	10
Apples			
fresh or frozen	Sainsbury	46	1 med/5oz 65
stewed (canned)	Tesco	67	19
stewed (unsweetened)	Sainsbury	35	1 tbsp/1oz 10
Apricot and almond yoghurt	St Michael	108	31
Apricot butter sponge pudding (as sold)	Tiffany's	195	$\frac{1}{4}$ pudding 150
Apricot conserve	BHS	260	74
Apricot date bar	Granose	246	70
Apricot Double Decker	St Michael	124	35
Apricot jam	Chivers		
	Extra	225	64
	Hartley's	260	74
	Robertson's	251	71
	Safeway	261	74
	Tesco	279	79

6

Product	Brand	Calories per 100g/ 100ml	Calories per oz/ pack/ portion
Apricot jam	Tesco Extra	268	76
	Waitrose	261	74
Apricot jam roll	Tesco	408	116
Apricot madeleines	Lyons	341	per cake 114
Apricot pie individual	Sainsbury Harvest (Lyons)	¼ pie 260 327	per pie 360
Apricot pie filling	Sainsbury	115	1 tbsp/2oz 65
	Tesco	82	23
Apricot preserve	Baxters	253	12oz/240g jar 860
Today's Recipe	Robertson's	180	51
Apricot roll	St Michael	359	102
Apricot slices	St Michael	335	per slice 251
Apricot Swiss roll (large)	Waitrose	317	90
Apricot tarts	Sainsbury		per tart 275
Apricot yoghurt	Waitrose	95	27
Apricots, canned		*106*	*30*
Apricots, canned	Libby	69	20
drained	Tesco	71	20
halves	Waitrose	106	30
halves in fruit juice	John West	40	11
Apricots, dried			
raw		*182*	*52*
stewed with sugar		*81*	*23*
stewed without sugar		*66*	*19*
Apricots, dried	Sainsbury	176	4 halves/ 1oz 50

Product	Brand	Calories per 100g/ 100ml	Calories per oz/ pack/ portion
Apricots, dried	Whitworths	166	47
ready cooked	Whitworths	164	46
Apricots, fresh			
raw		28	8
raw (with stones)		25	7
stewed with sugar		60	17
stewed with sugar (with stones)		57	16
stewed without sugar		23	6.5
stewed without sugar (with stones)		21	6
Apricots, fresh or frozen	Sainsbury	26	1×2oz 15
Arctic gâteau	Birds Eye		1/5 roll 100
Arctic log	Birds Eye		1/6 log 100
Arctic roll (small)	Birds Eye		1/6 roll 75
Aromat	Knorr	153	43
Arrabbiata Italian sauce	Homepride	126	376g pack 475
Arrow bars (all flavours)		381	108
Arrowroot		355	101
Artichokes, globe			
boiled		15	4.5
boiled (as served)		7	2
Artichokes, Jerusalem (boiled)		18	5
Asparagus, boiled		18	5
boiled (as served)		9	2.5
Asparagus, canned	Green Giant	15	4.5
	Libby	22	6

8

Product	Brand	Calories per 100g/ 100ml	Calories per oz/ pack/ portion
Asparagus, fresh, frozen or canned and drained	Sainsbury	35	1 tbsp/1oz 10
Asparagus soup *see also Cream of asparagus*			
	Batchelors	412	per portion 99
	Cup-a-Soup		per pack 224
	Batchelors		per portion 99
	5 Minute		per pack 224
condensed (undiluted)	Campbell's	72	20
dried (as sold)	Knorr	344	103
(made up)	Sainsbury	35	½ pint 100
Assorted biscuits	Waitrose	880	158
Assorted cream biscuits	Waitrose	500	142
Assorted meats	BHS		
cervelat		427	121
mortadella		219	62
smoked ham		157	44
tongue sausage		254	72
Assorted sweet biscuits	Sainsbury		per biscuit 55
Assorted wafers	Chiltonian	470	per wafer 40
Assorted whirls	Parkinsons	381	108
Aubergine, raw		*14*	*4*
Autumn Gold cider (bottled and canned)	Taunton	34	1 pint 200
Avocado pear		*223*	*63*
Avocado pear	Sainsbury	226	½ medium/ 5oz 320

Product	Brand	Calories per 100g/100ml	Calories per oz/pack/portion
Baby Bel cheese	Sainsbury	282	80
BACON *see also Gammon, etc*			
back	Waitrose	469	133
back rashers, raw	Danepak	370	105
Canadian style	St Michael	400	113
Danish smoked	St Michael	342	97
Danish unsmoked	St Michael	362	103
fried (average)		*465*	*132*
grilled (average)		*405*	*115*
grilled	Sainsbury		per rasher 65
mild cure	St Michael	395	112
raw		*428*	*121*
unsmoked	St Michael	390	111
collar joint, boiled, lean and fat		*325*	*92*
boiled, lean only		*191*	*54*
raw, lean and fat		*319*	*90*
Danish gammon D-shaped joint	St Michael	206	58
Danish smoked cured pork loin joint	St Michael	140	40
dressed carcase, raw		*352*	*100*
family rashers, raw	Danepack	260	74
fat, cooked (average)		*692*	*196*
raw (average)		*747*	*212*
fried rashers, lean only (average)		*332*	*94*
gammon	Waitrose	324	92
boiled lean	Sainsbury	176	50
gammon joint, boiled, lean and fat		*269*	*76*

Product	Brand	Calories per 100g/ 100ml	Calories per oz/ pack/ portion
BACON, gammon joint			
boiled, lean only		167	47
raw, lean and fat		236	67
gammon rashers,			
grilled, lean and fat		228	65
grilled, lean only		172	49
gammon steaks,			
Canadian style	St Michael	182	52
Danish D-shaped	St Michael	206	58
Danish round			
unsmoked	St Michael	173	49
grilled rashers,			
lean only (average)		292	83
half gammon			
rashers, unsmoked	St Michael	234	66
hock	Waitrose	356	101
lean, raw (average)		147	42
middle rashers, 200g			
pack (uncooked)	Danepak	400	113
fried (average)		477	135
grilled (average)		416	118
grilled	Sainsbury		per rasher 65
raw		425	120
mildcure joint	St Michael	198	56
rind-on gammon			
joint, smoked	St Michael	246	70
steaks, raw	Danepak	180	51
streaky	Waitrose	508	144
streaky rashers, raw	Danepak	450	128

11

Product	Brand	Calories per 100g/ 100ml	Calories per oz/ pack/ portion
BACON, streaky rashers			
Canadian style	St Michael	410	116
fried (average)		496	141
grilled (average)		422	120
grilled	Sainsbury		per rasher 45
raw		414	117
unsmoked	St Michael	400	113
Bacon, cheese and egg pie	Sainsbury	317	¼ pie/3oz 270
Bacon, mushroom and peppers pizza	St Michael	182	52
Bacon and egg pie	Sainsbury	378	¼ pie/2oz 215
Bacon and ham loaf	Sainsbury	212	60
Bacon and liver sausage	Sainsbury	212	60
Bacon Bites	Danish Prime	285	81
	Tesco	491	139
Bacon burgers	Danish Prime	275	78
Bacon fingers	Danish Prime	240	68
Bacon puffs	Tesco	491	139
Bacon savoury mash	Yeoman	371	per portion made up 69
Bacon Streaks	Safeway	451	129
Baked Alaska	St Michael	266	75
Baked beans	BHS	79	22
	Sainsbury	88	1tbsp/1oz 25
	Waitrose	92	26
and frankfurters	Sainsbury	127	7¾oz can 280
and hamburgers	Sainsbury	123	7¾oz can 270
and sausages	Sainsbury	155	7¾oz can 340

Product	Brand	Calories per 100g/ 100ml	Calories per oz/ pack/ portion
Baked beans			
with hamburgers	Chef	122	35
with pork sausages	Chef	124	35
	Heinz	126	36
with tomato sauce	Armour	64	18
	Crosse & Blackwell	96	27
	Heinz	72	20
Bakewell creams	Tesco	485	137
Bakewell tart	BHS	416	303g tart 1260
	Sainsbury	414	1/5 tart/2oz 235
Baking powder		*163*	*46*
Baking powder	Tesco	130	37
Banana bar	Palm	400	113
	Prewetts	182	per bar 76
Banana blancmange (as sold)	Brown & Polson	324	92
Banana Delight (made up)	Tesco	134	38
Banana dessert	Waitrose	46	13
Banana ice-cream, family brick	Lyons Maid		per pack 401
Banana lolly	Lyons Maid		per lolly 46
Banana Munch Bunch	Eden Vale	102	29
Banana supreme dessert	Sainsbury		pkt made up 450
Banana Two Shakes	Kellogg's	360 (100g dry)	1/2 sachet (20g) + 1/2 pint milk 273

13

Product	Brand	Calories per 100g/ 100ml	Calories per oz/ pack/ portion
Banana yogurt/ yoghurt	Eden Vale	92	26
	Sainsbury	102	sm. tub/¼ pint 145
	Ski	96	27
	Waitrose	95	27
Bananas, raw (with skin)		79	22
		47	13
Bananas, raw	Sainsbury	47	1 med./6oz 80
Bandit	McVitie		per biscuit 103
Banjo,			
coconut funsize	Mars		each 80
coconut single			each 114
peanut funsize	Mars		each 80
peanut single			each 119
Bar 6	Cadbury's	543	154
Bar gâteau	BHS	343	97
Barbary biscuits	Huntley & Palmers	511	per biscuit 51
Barbecue and onion crisps	St Michael	533	151
Barbecue beef and tomato soup	Batchelors 5-Minute		per pack 171
Barbecue Coat & Cook	Homepride	395	43g pack 170
Barbecue Cook-in-Sauce	Homepride	76	376g pack 285
Barbecue sauce mix (as sold)	Colman's	310	88
	Knorr	349	99
Barbecue sticks	St Michael	485	137
Barcelona nuts (with shells)		639	181
		396	112

14

Product	Brand	Calories per 100g/ 100ml	Calories per oz/ pack/ portion
Barley, pearl			
boiled		120	34
raw		360	102
Barley, pearl	Safeway	360	102
	Sainsbury	353	100 raw
		123	35 cooked
	Tesco	357	101
	Waitrose	360	102
	Whitworths	360	102 raw
		120	34 cooked
Barley sugar	Barker & Dobson Callard and Bowser,	320	91
	Nuttall	380	per sweet 24
golden	Pascall	376	107
old fashioned	Parkinsons	378	107
Basil, rubbed	Tesco	250	71
Basmati rice (raw)	Whitworths	363	103
Bath buns	Sainsbury		per bun 165
	St Michael	419	119
Bath Oliver biscuits	Fortts	440	per biscuit 49
Battenberg cake	Lyons	366	per cake 1072
	Sainsbury	364	1/8 cake/ 1½ oz 155
	BHS	342	per cake 941
	St Michael	360	102
	Waitrose	370	105
Batter mix, quick (as sold)	Whitworths	338	500g pack 1690

Product	Brand	Calories per 100g/ 100ml	Calories per oz/ pack/ portion
Bavarian Brie:	Tesco		
blue with herbs &			
peppers		434	123
with green peppercorns		432	122
Bavarian ham			
sausage	St Michael	160	45
Bavarian processed			
cheese	Tesco	310	88
with ham	Tesco	300	85
Bavarian salad	Eden Vale	162	46
Bavarian smoked			
cheese	Sainsbury	282	1in cube/ 1oz 80
	Tesco	310	88
with ham	Tesco	300	85
Bay leaves	Tesco	300	85
Beans *see also Butter Beans, Cannelloni, etc*			
Beans, raw	Safeway	15	4.5
cooked		7	2
large, dried	Surprise	270	per pack 89
whole	St Michael	35	10
Beans and pork			
sausages in tomato			
sauce	Tesco	123	35
Beans in tomato sauce	Tesco	105	30
Beansprouts, canned		9	2.5
Bearnaise Master			
Sauce (as sold)	Colman's	365	103
BEEF			
braising	St Michael	128	36

Product	Brand	Calories per 100g/ 100ml	Calories per oz/ pack/ portion
BEEF			
brisket, boiled, lean and fat		326	92
raw, lean and fat		252	71
corned, canned		217	62
dressed carcase, raw		282	80
fat,			
cooked (average)		613	174
raw (average)		637	181
flash fry	St Michael	128	36
forerib,			
raw, lean and fat		290	82
roast, lean and fat		349	99
roast, lean only		225	64
ground	St Michael	128	36
lean, raw (average)		123	35
mince	St Michael	321	91
cooked without fat	Sainsbury	229	1tbsp/1oz 65
raw		221	63
stewed		229	65
rib eye joint	St Michael	176	50
rump	St Michael	123	35
rump steak			
fried, lean and fat		246	70
fried, lean only		190	54
grilled, lean and fat		218	62
grilled, lean only		168	48
raw, lean and fat		197	56
silverside, salted,			
boiled, lean and fat		242	69

Product	Brand	Calories per 100g/ 100ml	Calories per oz/ pack/ portion
BEEF, silverside			
salted, boiled, lean only		173	49
joint, cured	St Michael	242	69
sirloin, cooked	Sainsbury	194	1 slice/2oz lean 110
raw, lean and fat		272	77
roast, lean and fat		284	81
roast, lean only		192	54
thin cut	St Michael	116	33
stewing	St Michael	128	36
cooked	Sainsbury	212	1tbsp/2oz lean only 120
raw, lean and fat		176	50
stewed, lean and fat		223	63
top rump joint	St Michael	179	51
topside	St Michael	179	51
cooked	Sainsbury	159	1 slice/2oz lean only 90
raw, lean and fat		179	51
roast, lean and fat		214	61
roast, lean only		156	44
tournedos (20% pork fat)	St Michael	158	45
Beef, cheese and tomato croquettes, sizzle	Tiffany's	225	per croquette 117
Beef and bacon paste	Princes	234	66
Beef and gravy	Batchelors	119	per can 495
Beef and kidney	Batchelors	94	per can 392

18

Product	Brand	Calories per 100g/ 100ml	Calories per oz/ pack/ portion
Beef and mushroom paste	St Michael	262	74
Beef and onion	Batchelors	122	per can 508
Beef and onion flavour potato snacks	Sainsbury	560	140
Beef and onion paste	St Michael	262	74
Beef and onion pie (fresh)	Tesco	277	79
Beef and onion slice, farmhouse	Kraft	340	each (113g) 385
Beef and onion soup (as sold)	Knorr Quick	355	101
Beef and pork sausage meat	Sainsbury	353	100
Beef and potato pasties (284g)	BHS	281	per pack 799
Beef and tomato soup	Batchelors		
	Cup-a-Soup	341	per portion 58
	Slim-a-Soup	292	per portion 35
Beef and tomato Pot Noodle	Golden Wonder		carton made up 370
Beef and vegetable extract cubes	Safeway	238	68
Beef and vegetable pie 4½oz oval, baked	Tiffany's	255	per pie 295
340g/12oz	Kraft	270	each 920
1lb, baked	Tiffany's	245	¼ pie 280
frozen	Tesco	280	79
individual	Ross	280	79

19

Product	Brand	Calories per 100g/ 100ml	Calories per oz/ pack/ portion
Beef and vegetable pudding	Sainsbury	162	5oz 230
Beef and vegetable slice (fresh)	Tesco	277	79
Beef and vegetable soup	Heinz Big Soups	53	15
condensed (undiluted)	Campbell's Main-Course	70	20
Beef biriani	Vesta	381	per pack 690
Beef Bites	Sainsbury	500	25g 125
Beef bourguignon Casserole Mix (as sold)	Colman's	350	99
Beef broth	Heinz Big Soups	55	16
	Heinz Ready to Serve	41	12
condensed (undiluted)	Campbell's	83	24
Scotch	Baxters	41	15oz/425g can 171
Beef casserole (425g)	Goblin	100	per pack 425
(ready meal)	Ross	70	20
Beef chipolatas	Tesco	320	91
	Waitrose	289	82
Beef chow mein	Snackpot	347	per pot 205
Beef croquettes, sizzle	Tiffany's	250	each 145
Beef curry, condensed (undiluted)	Campbell's Today's Special	162	50

Product	Brand	Calories per 100g/ 100ml	Calories per oz/ pack/ portion
Beef curry			
hot	Vesta	362	per pack 822
and rice (ready meal)	Ross	150	43
with rice	Birds Eye		per pack 380
with separate rice	Crosse & Blackwell	125	35
Beef dripping		891	*253*
Beef dripping	Tesco	931	264
Beef flavour soup	Chef Chunky	57	16
Beef flavour and vegetable soup (made up)	Chef Box	25	7
Beef goulash (Cook in the Pot)	Crosse & Blackwell	380	108
Beef grills	Ross	330	94
Beef loaf	St Michael	260	74
lean beef	Sainsbury	159	1 thin slice/ 1oz 45
Beef paste	Shippams	205	58
with pickle	Country Pot	160	45
with tomato	Country Pot	145	41
Beef pie, family	Ross	270	77
value	Birds Eye		each 370
Beef Provençale mix (as sold)	Colman's	280	79
Beef risotto	Snackpot	291	per pot 201
	Vesta	363	per pack 625
Beef sausages	Safeway	262	75
	Sainsbury	203 grilled	1, 2oz grilled 115

21

Product	Brand	Calories per 100g/ 100ml	Calories per oz/ pack/ portion
Beef sausages	Sainsbury	282 raw	1, 2oz, raw 160
	St Michael	341	97
	Waitrose	289	82
(12 per pack)	BHS	395	113
(8 per pack)	Tesco	322	91
skinless	Sainsbury	212 grilled	1, 1oz, 60 grilled
		282 raw	1, 1oz, 80 raw
	Waitrose	289	82
Beef seasoning (as sold)	Colman's	315	89
Beef soup, canned	Heinz	64	18
	Sainsbury	35	½ pint 100
Beef spread	Princes	212	60
	St Michael	300	85
Beef steak pie, topcrust	St Michael	203	58
with onion	St Michael	271	77
Beef steak pudding, cooked		223	63
Beef stew		119	34
Beef stew	Campbell's	77	22
and dumpling	Birds Eye		per pack 240
Beef stock see also Oxo condensed			
(undiluted)	Campbell's	88	25
	Fray Bentos	220	62
cubes	Beecham	259	73
	Knorr	314	9.5g cube 30

Product	Brand	Calories per 100g/ 100ml	Calories per oz/ pack/ portion
Beef stock			
powder	Knorr	171	85g pack 145
tablets	Safeway	240	69
Beef stroganoff (Cook in the Pot)	Crosse & Blackwell	418	118
Beef stroganoff, Casserole mix (as sold)	Colman's	320	91
Beefburgers *see also* **Beefburgers**	Danish		
Beefburgers	Prime	255	72
(4×2oz)	Tiffany's	264	each 149
(10/24×1¾oz)	Tiffany's	264	each 132
all beef (2oz)	Sainsbury	238	each 135
(4oz)		247	each 280
(6oz)		235	each 400
American style	St Michael	258	73
Beefburgers, frozen			
fried		264	75
raw		265	75
Beefburgers, frozen	Ross	270	77
	Sainsbury	247	140
	Waitrose	176	50
100% beef	Birds Eye		each, grilled or fried 120
	Ross	320	91
quarter pounders	Birds Eye		each, grilled 260, fried 290
with or without onions	Tesco	157	45
Beefburgers, quarter pounders	Tiffany's	264	each 298
in gravy	Tesco	145	41

23

Product	Brand	Calories per 100g/ 100ml	Calories per oz/ pack/ portion
Beefburgers			
with onion	Brains		per burger well grilled 80
	Kraft		per burger well grilled 80
	St Michael	260	74
fresh	Tesco	237	67
frozen, with onion	Birds Eye		each, grilled or fried 130
Beefburgers with onions and gravy (411g)	Goblin	140	per pack 575
Beefburgers without onion	St Michael	260	74
fresh	Tesco	313	89
Beefsteak pie, family	Brains		per pie 1680
Beefy drink	Safeway	176	50
Beer			
bitter, canned		*32*	*9*
bitter, draught		*32*	*9*
bitter, keg		*31*	*9*
brown ale, bottled		*28*	*8*
lager	Sainsbury	28	½ pint 80
lager, bottled		*29*	*8*
mild, draught		*25*	*7*
pale ale, bottled		*32*	*9*
stout, bottled		*37*	*10*
stout, extra		*39*	*11*
strong ale		*72*	*20*
Beer shandy	Minster	25	7
Beetroot			
boiled		*44*	*12*
raw		*28*	*8*

24

Product	Brand	Calories per 100g/ 100ml	Calories per oz/ pack/ portion
Beetroot, all			
varieties	Haywards	40	11
fresh	Sainsbury	53	1 tbsp/1oz 15
Beetroot, pickled	Safeway	44	13
baby	Baxters	45	12oz/340g jar 153
	BHS	30	8.5
	Waitrose	46	13
sliced	Baxters	30	11¾oz/333g jar 102 20oz/567g jar 170 40oz/1134g jar 340
	BHS	30	8.5
sliced or whole	Epicure	29	8
	St Michael	44	13
	Tesco	39	11
sweet sliced	Epicure	46	13
Beetroot and redcurrant relish	Baxters	169	8oz/227g jar 383
Beetroot in vinaigrette	St Michael	165	47
Beetroot salad	Sainsbury	88	1 tbsp/1oz 25
canned	Tesco	137	39
Bemax		347	98
Bemax	Beecham Foods	350	99
crunchy	Beecham Foods	324	92
Bengal gram see Chick peas			

25

Product	Brand	Calories per 100g/ 100ml	Calories per oz/ pack/ portion
Bicarbonate of soda	Whitworths	nil	
Bierwurst	BHS	314	89
	St Michael	200	57
Big Country rolls,			
brown	St Michael	261	74
soft	St Michael	268	76
white	St Michael	271	77
Big Country white bread	St Michael	258	73
Big Dipper (straw./van.)	Wall's		each 110
Big Feast	Wall's		each 232
Big Value mash	Yeoman	331 (dry)	per portion made up 61
Bigtop biscuits:	Chiltonian		
chocolate		465	per biscuit 18
coconut		496	per biscuit 19
lemon and lime		500	per biscuit 19
vanilla		480	per biscuit 19
Bilberries, raw		*56*	*16*
Biscuits *see also under names – Club, Digestive, etc*			
Biscuits			
home-made		*469*	*133*
semi-sweet		*457*	*130*
short-sweet		*469*	*133*
Biscuits for cheese	BHS	527	149
Biskwheat cereal	Safeway	351	100
Bitter lemon	Waitrose	34	9.5
Bitter lemon (bottled)	Club	26	113ml 30 185ml 50

Product	Brand	Calories per 100g/ 100ml	Calories per oz/ pack/ portion
Bitter lemon (bottled)	Safeway	20–30	6–9
	Sainsbury	32	125ml/¼ pint 45
	Tesco	33	9.5
Bitter lemon, low calorie (bottled)	Club	negl.	113ml, 185ml, negl.
	Sainsbury	3.5	125ml/¼ pint 5
	Tesco	6	2
Bitter lemon, Slimline	Schweppes	1.7	
Bitter lemon, sparkling	Schweppes	32	9
Bitter lemon crush	Britvic	46	13
	Slimsta	5	1.5
Bitter lemon drink, bittersweet low calorie sparkling (canned)	Hunts	5	1.5
Bitter lemon drink, low calorie (bottled)	Hunts	4	1
Bitter lemon drink, sparkling (bottled)	Hunts	33	9.5
	Idris	34	9.5
Bitter lemon drink, sparkling (canned)	Hunts	34	9.5
Bitter lemon sandwich biscuits	Sainsbury		per biscuit 65
Bitter orange drink, low calorie sparkling (bottled)	Hunts	5	1.5

Product	Brand	Calories per 100g/ 100ml	Calories per oz/ pack/ portion
Black cherry and buttercream roll	Sainsbury	329	¹/₆ roll/ 1½oz 140
Black cherry cheesecake mix (as sold)	Whitworths	430	11oz pack 1339
Black cherry conserve	BHS	260	74
Black cherry Double Decker	St Michael	124	35
Black cherry jam	Chivers		
	Extra	220	62
	Hartley's	225	64
	Waitrose	261	74
Black cherry jam, extra	Tesco	268	76
Black cherry ripple, cutting brick	Lyons Maid		per pack 909
family brick	Lyons Maid		per pack 432
Black cherry yogurt/ yoghurt	BHS	80	150g pack 120
	Sainsbury	123	¼ pint tub 175
	St Michael	97	27
	Ski	94	27
	Waitrose	95	27
Black Forest gâteau	Ross	300	85
	St Michael	278	79
Black Jacks	Trebor		per sweet 14
Black pepper, ground	Whitworths	324	92
ground or whole	Tesco	275	78
Black pudding (fried)		*305*	*86*
Black pudding	Sainsbury	229	65
	John West	312	88

28

product	Brand	Calories per 100g/ 100ml	Calories per oz/ pack/ portion
Blackberries			
raw		29	8
stewed with sugar		60	17
stewed without sugar		25	7
Blackberries			
canned (inc. syrup)	Sainsbury	97	1 tbsp/1oz 27
fresh or frozen	Sainsbury	31	1 tbsp/1oz 9
frozen	Waitrose	28	8
Blackberry and apple rumble	Sainsbury	163	¼ pack/ 4oz 185
Blackberry and apple pie filling	Waitrose	77	22
Blackberry Munch Bunch	Eden Vale	105	30
Blackcurrant and apple pie (4 portion)	Sainsbury		¼ pie 250
Blackcurrant cheesecake	St Michael	263	75
Blackcurrant cheesecake mix (as sold)	Whitworths	430	11oz pack 1339
Blackcurrant conserve	BHS	260	74
Blackcurrant crush	Slimsta	2.5	0.7
sparkling	Waitrose	34	9.5
Blackcurrant drink	BHS	39	11
	Cresta	33	9.5
	Sainsbury	44	½ pint diluted from 4 tbsp 125

Product	Brand	Calories per 100g/ 100ml	Calories per oz/ pack/ portion
Blackcurrant drink concentrated (undiluted)	Waitrose	220	65
	Tesco	95	27
Blackcurrant flan filling	Armour	100	28
Blackcurrant flavour cordial (undiluted)	Britvic	124	35
	Corona	130	37
	Idris	130	37
	Schweppes	135	38
Blackcurrant health drink (511ml/18fl.oz)	BHS	282	per pack 144
Blackcurrant jam	Chivers		
	Extra	240	68
	Hartley's	250	71
	Moorhouse	255	72
	Robertson's	251	71
	Safeway	261	74
	Tesco	279	79
	Tesco Extra	268	76
	Waitrose	261	74
Blackcurrant jelly (dessert), as sold	Chivers	260	74
	Waitrose	258	73
Blackcurrant jelly (preserve)	Hartley's	255	72
Blackcurrant pie	Waitrose	190	54
Blackcurrant pie filling	Pack-a-Pie	61	per pack 249
	Sainsbury	141	1 tbsp/2oz 80
	Waitrose	102	29

Product	Brand	Calories per 100g/ 100ml	Calories per oz/ pack/ portion
Blackcurrant preserve	Baxters	260	12oz/340g jar 884
Today's Recipe	Robertson's	180	51
Blackcurrant Rise and Shine	Kellogg's	337 (dry)	4fl.oz/114ml 50
Blackcurrant roll	St Michael	353	100
Blackcurrant Royale	St Ivel	125	35
Blackcurrant split (288g)	Wall's	155	per pack 445
Blackcurrant sponge roll	Lyons	357	per roll 978
Blackcurrant sundaes	Sainsbury		per cake 190
	St Michael	413	per cake 204
Blackcurrant tarts	Sainsbury		per tart 290
Blackcurrant yoghurt	Waitrose	95	27
Blackcurrants, canned (inc. syrup)	Hartley's	85	24
	Sainsbury	97	1 tbsp/1oz 27
frozen	Waitrose	28	8
Blackcurrants, raw		28	8
stewed with sugar		59	17
stewed without sugar		24	7
Blackforest gâteau	Birds Eye		⅙ cake 250
Blackthorn cider	Taunton	34	1 pint 200
Blancmange (Brown & Polson) *see under flavours*			
Blancmange (mix), made up	Sainsbury	119	34
Bloater, grilled		251	71
(with bones)		186	53
Bloater paste	Shippams	140	40

Product	Brand	Calories per 100g/ 100ml	Calories per oz/ pack/ portion
Bloomer, large and small	St Michael	250	71
Blue Riband	Rowntree Mackintosh	530	150
Blueberry pie filling	Pack-a-Pie	62	per pack 253
Bockwurst	St Michael	280	79
Boil in the bag rice (raw)	Kellogg's	327	93
Boiled sweets		*327*	*93*
Boiled sweets	Trebor		per sweet 25
Bologna	Granose	167	47
Bolognaise sauce	Tesco	100	28
Pour Over	Crosse & Blackwell	70	20
Bolognese (as sold)	Beanfeast	291	per pack 334
Bolognese sauce		*139*	*39*
	Buitoni	51	14
	Campbell's Spaghetti Sauces	101	29
	Granose	60	17
undiluted	Campbell's Prego	100	28
Bombay chicken curry Knoodles	Knorr	369	105
Bon bons (bag)	Sharps		per pack 480 per sweet 26
Border creme eggs	Cadbury's	434	123
Borderline Master Sauce (as sold)	Colman's	335	95

Product	Brand	Calories per 100g/ 100ml	Calories per oz/ pack/ portion
Boston pickle	Crosse & Blackwell	107	30
Bounty		*473*	*134*
Bounty:	Mars		
funsize			each 150
milk single			each 150
plain single			each 147
Bourbon biscuits	Peek Frean	466	per biscuit 60
	Sainsbury		per biscuit 65
Bourbon creams	BHS	466	132
	Pennywise		per biscuit 54
	Tesco	487	138
Bournville assorted biscuits:	Cadbury's		
barrel		500	142
ring		480	136
sandwich		500	142
triangle		475	135
wafer		510	145
Bourneville chocolate bar	Cadbury's	513	145
fruit and nut		464	132
roasted almond		534	151
Bourneville cocoa	Cadbury's	455	129
Bourneville Selection chocolates	Cadbury's	466	132
Bournvita		*377*	*107*
Bournvita	Cadbury's	380	108
Bovril		*174*	*49*
Bovril	Beecham	189	54
cubes		259	73

33

Product	Brand	Calories per 100g/100ml	Calories per oz/pack/portion
Braemar biscuits	Huntley & Palmers	469	per biscuit 49
Brain			
calf, boiled		152	43
calf and lamb, raw		110	31
lamb, boiled		126	36
Braised kidneys and gravy	Birds Eye		per pack 200
Bramble jam, seedless	Moorhouse	265	75
Bramble jelly	Hartley's	260	74
wild	Baxters	260	12oz/340g jar 884
Bramley apple flan filling	Armour	77	22
Bramley apple pie filling	Sainsbury	70	1 tbsp/2oz 40
Bramley apple sauce	Pan Yan	115	33
Bramley apple tart	St Michael	223	63
Bran (wheat)		206	58
Bran, broad	Allinson	152	43
country	Jordans	293	83
farmhouse	Weetabix	303	86
fruit	Granose	302	86
natural	Granose	296	84
natural wheat	Prewetts	152	43
soya	Granose	230	65
toasted	Meadow Farm	350	100
toasted farmhouse	Weetabix	300	30g serving 90

Product	Brand	Calories per 100g/ 100ml	Calories per oz/ pack/ portion
Bran biscuits	Allinson	521	148
Bran bread mix	Allinson	361	102
Bran Buds	Kellogg's	254	72
Bran Fare	Weetabix	267	76
Bran Flakes	Kellogg's	315	89
Bran oatcakes	Allinson	419	119
Bran Plus cereal	Allinson	222	63
Bran Sunnywheat biscuits	St Michael	380	per biscuit 38
Brandy cake (canned)	Lyons	319	per cake 2622
Branston fruity pickle	Crosse & Blackwell	90	26
Branston pickle	Crosse & Blackwell	131	37
Branston spicy sauce	Crosse & Blackwell	112	32
Brawn		*153*	*43*
Brawn	Sainsbury	194	1 thin slice/ 1oz 55
Brazil kernels	Sainsbury	635	180
Brazil nuts (with shells)		*619* *277*	*175* *79*
Brazil nuts	Whitworths	619	175
Brazil nuts, roasted	Tesco	800	227
Brazil nut toffees	Callard & Bowser, Nuttall	480	per sweet 40
Brazilian mix	Prewetts	407	115

Product	Brand	Calories per 100g/ 100ml	Calories per oz/ pack/ portion
BREAD			
brown		223	63
currant		250	71
fried		558	158
Hovis		228	65
malt		248	70
soda		264	75
toasted		297	84
white		233	66
wholemeal		216	61
BREAD, BRANDED LOAVES			
Allinson	St Michael	215	61
Big Country white bloomer, large or small	St Michael	258	73
Coburg	St Michael	250	71
country bran	St Michael	236	67
cracked wheat	St Michael	222	63
farmhouse crusty	St Michael	250	71
granary	St Michael	237	67
Hovis	St Michael	230	65
mixed grain	St Michael	225	64
Old English	St Michael	241	68
split tin crusty	St Michael	250	71
square loaf	St Michael	237	67
stick, crusty toasting, small	St Michael	250	71
white	St Michael	269	76
Vitbe	St Michael	240	68
white	Sainsbury		thin slice 70 medium slice 95

36

Product	Brand	Calories per 100g/ 100ml	Calories per oz/ pack/ portion
BREAD, BRANDED LOAVES, white			
	Sainsbury		thick slice 115
white sliced (medium or thin)	St Michael	228	65
wholemeal	Sainsbury		thin slice 65 medium slice 85 thick slice 110
Bread and butter pudding		*159*	*45*
Bread mix, bran	Allinson	361	102
everready	Prewetts	334	95
white	Allinson	351	100
wholewheat	Allinson	329	93
BREAD ROLLS			
brown, crusty		*289*	*82*
brown, soft		*282*	*80*
starch reduced		*384*	*109*
white, crusty		*290*	*82*
white, soft		*305*	*86*
BREAD ROLLS, BRANDED			
Aberdeen	St Michael	421	119
Big Country brown	St Michael	261	74
Big Country soft	St Michael	268	76
Big Country white	St Michael	271	77
breakfast, packs of 4 or 6	St Michael	254	72
crisp	St Michael	375	per roll 38
mixed grain	St Michael	224	64
Old English	St Michael	278	79
wheatmeal	Granose	349	99

Product	Brand	Calories per 100g/ 100ml	Calories per oz/ pack/ portion
BREAD ROLLS, BRANDED			
white	Granose	356	101
white, ready to bake	St Michael	271	77
Bread sauce		*110*	*31*
Bread sauce mix	Colman's	320	91
(as sold)	Knorr	361	102
	Whitworths	340	96
(made up)	Chef Box	105	30
	Sainsbury	106	1 tbsp/1oz 30
Breadcrumbs, dried		*354*	*100*
Breadcrumbs, golden	Tesco	348	99
Breakaway, milk	Rowntree Mackintosh	515	146
Breakfast cereal	Waitrose	384	109
Breakfast oats	Prewetts	405	115
Breakfast rolls, packs of 4 or 6	St Michael	254	72
Breakfast slice, grilled	Sainsbury		per slice 75
Break In biscuits	St Michael	590	each 119
Breast of chicken roll	Ross	150	43
Breast of turkey	Ross	140	40
Breton pâté	BHS	397	113
Brie *see also Bavarian Brie*			
Brie	BHS	307	87
	Sainsbury	265	75
	St Ivel	295	84
	St Michael	297	84
	Tesco	307	87
blue	BHS	463	131

product	Brand	Calories per 100g/ 100ml	Calories per oz/ pack/ portion
Brisket see Beef			
Britvic 55			
grapefruit		51	14
orange		52	15
pineapple		53	15
Broad beans, canned	Hartley's	100	28
	Sainsbury	35	1 tbsp/1oz 10
	Waitrose	42	12
canned, drained	Tesco	49	14
fresh, frozen or			
canned and drained	Sainsbury	35	10
frozen	Birds Eye	53	15
	Ross	70	20
	St Michael	48	14
Broad bran	Allinson	152	43
Broccoli (tops), boiled		*18*	*5*
raw		*23*	*6.5*
Broccoli, fresh or frozen	Sainsbury	18	1–2 spears/ 1oz 5
frozen	Waitrose	32	9
stir fry	St Michael	29	8
Broccoli spears, frozen	Birds Eye	35	10
	BHS	25	225g pack 56
	Ross	25	7
Broth see also brand names or flavours			
Broth, bone and vegetable		*60*	*17*
Brown ale, bottled		*28*	*8*
Brown bread		*223*	*63*

Product	Brand	Calories per 100g/ 100ml	Calories per oz/ pack/ portion
Brown crystal sugar	Tesco	394	112
Brown rice (raw)	Whitworths	360	102
Brown sauce (bottled)		*99*	*28*
Brown sauce	Sainsbury	53	1 tbsp/1oz 15
catering pack	Pan Yan	185	52
Browning	Crosse & Blackwell	195	55
Brunchies	Birds Eye		each, grilled 155, fried 180
Brussels sprouts, boiled		*18*	*5*
raw		*26*	*7.5*
Brussels sprouts, fresh, frozen or canned and drained	Sainsbury	35	3 sprouts/1oz 10
frozen	BHS	40	11
	Ross	40	11
	Tesco	35	10
	Waitrose	32	9
Bubble and squeak (as sold)	Ross	70	20
Bubble ball	Lyons Maid		each 101
Bubble 'n' squeak	Birds Eye		per patty grilled 85 fried 175
Buccatini	St Michael	472	134
Bulmers Conditioned Draught cider:	H.P. Bulmer		
dry		27	7.5
medium		29	8
sweet		34	9.5

Product	Brand	Calories per 100g/ 100ml	Calories per oz/ pack/ portion
Bunnytots	Rowntree Mackintosh	420	sm. bag 170
Buns *see Bath, Round, etc*			
Burford biscuits	Huntley & Palmers	447	per biscuit 60
Burgers *see also Beefburgers, Hamburgers*			
Burgers, chuck steak	St Michael	218	62
quarter pounders	St Michael	245	69
value	Birds Eye		each, grilled 95, fried 115
Burgundy wine Cooking-In sauce	Baxters	49	425g can 209
Butter (salted)		*740*	*210*
Butter	Safeway	795	226
	Sainsbury	776	1 tbsp/½oz 110
	St Ivel	735	208
	Tesco	775	220
blended dairy	Waitrose	797	226
Cornish	Waitrose	797	226
Dutch	Waitrose	797	226
English roll	St Michael	793	225
French	Waitrose	797	226
Irish	Waitrose	797	226
New Zealand	Waitrose	797	226
Welsh	Waitrose	797	226
Butter beans, raw		*273*	*77*
boiled		*95*	*27*
Butter beans, canned	Batchelors	68	19
	Hartley's	95	27
canned, drained	Sainsbury	88	1 tbsp/1oz 25
	Tesco	95	27

41

Product	Brand	Calories per 100g/ 100ml	Calories per oz/ pack/ portion
Butter beans			
canned, drained	Waitrose	98	28
dried, raw	Safeway	266	76
	Sainsbury	265	75
cooked		106	30
dried, raw	Waitrose	268	76
	Whitworths	273	77
cooked		95	27
Butter Crinkle	BHS	457	130
biscuits	Safeway	457	130
Butter Crunch	St Michael	463	per biscuit 33
biscuits	Waitrose	455	129
Butter Crunch creams	St Michael	503	per biscuit 67
Butter mints	Sainsbury	370	105
Butter Osborne			
biscuits	Peek Frean	437	per biscuit 35
Butter puffs	Crawfords		per biscuit 50
	St Michael	503	per biscuit 50
Butter rings	Tesco	533	151
Butter Shorties	Safeway	493	141
Butter sultana			
cookies	Sainsbury		per biscuit 65
Butter toffee			
bon-bons	St Michael	380	108
Butter walnut	Sainsbury	364	1/6 cake/1½oz
sandwich			155
Buttercrisp biscuits	Jacobs	460	per biscuit 40
Butterdrops, old			
fashioned	Parkinsons	382	108
Buttermint thins	Parkinsons	420	119

42

Product	Brand	Calories per 100g/ 100ml	Calories per oz/ pack/ portion
Butterscotch	Parkinsons	420	119
	Pascall	412	117
	Sainsbury	388	110
	Tesco	425	120
100g pkt	Callard & Bowser, Nuttall	410	per sweet 34
stick, bag, box or loose	Callard & Bowser, Nuttall	410	per sweet 26
Butterscotch Delight (made up)	Tesco	134	38
Butterscotch dessert	Waitrose	465	132
Butterscotch dessert sauce	Lyons Maid	314	89
Butterscotch supreme dessert	Sainsbury		pkt made up 480
Buttons *see Chocolate buttons*			

Product	Brand	Calories per 100g/ 100ml	Calories per oz/ pack/ portion
Cabana	Rowntree Mackintosh	445	per pack 255
Cabbage			
red, raw		20	6
Savoy, boiled		9	2.5
Savoy, raw		26	7.5
spring, boiled		7	2
white, raw		22	6
winter, boiled		15	4.5
winter, raw		22	6
Cabbage, chopped	Birds Eye	21	6
fresh or frozen	Sainsbury	35	1tbsp/1oz 10
shredded	Ross	30	9
Cacciatora Italian sauce	Homepride	94	376g pack 355
Cadbury chocolate éclairs	Pascall	441	125
Cadbury's chocolate *see Dairy Milk, etc*			
Caerphilly cheese	Sainsbury	353	100
	Tesco	356	101
	Waitrose	356	101
Cakes *see Madeira, etc*			
Calf liver *see liver*			
Camembert cheese	BHS	303	86
	Sainsbury	300	85
	St Ivel	315	89
	St Michael	312	88
	Tesco	300	85
Candy cookies	Sainsbury		per biscuit 40
Candy sticks	Bassett's	406	115
Candy sugar	Tesco	394	112

44

Product	Brand	Calories per 100g/ 100ml	Calories per oz/ pack/ portion
Candytots	Rowntree Mackintosh	400	sm. bag 175
Cannellini beans	Batchelors	68	19
Cannelloni	Buitoni	97	27
	Crosse & Blackwell	103	29
frozen (396g)	BHS	89	per pack 352
Capon	Waitrose	120	34
Captain's Pie	Birds Eye	119	8oz pack 270
		121	14oz pack 480
Caramac	Rowntree Mackintosh	555	med. pack 155
Caramel bar	Cadbury's	488	149
Caramel blancmange (as sold)	Brown & Polson	324	31g pack 100
Caramel cookies	Tesco	516	146
Caramel Delight	St Michael	139	39
Caramel dessert	Sainsbury		pkt made up 800
	St Michael	135	38
Caramel dessert sauce	Tesco	320	91
Caramel dessert topping	Colman's	300	85
Caramel fudge	Lyons Maid		each 168
Caramel log	Tunnock's		per biscuit 121
Caramel shortcakes	Sainsbury		per cake 140
Caramel wafers	Sainsbury		per biscuit 85
	Tesco	476	135
	Tunnock's		per biscuit 120

Product	Brand	Calories per 100g/ 100ml	Calories per oz/ pack/ portion
Caramel wafers, milk	St Michael	493	per biscuit 96
milk chocolate	Sainsbury		per biscuit 125
Cariba	Schweppes	35	10
Caribbean drink (frozen)	St Michael	205	58
Caribbean fruit drink	St Michael	55	16
Caribbean salad	Eden Vale	130	37
Carob chip biscuits	Prewetts	524	149
Carob fruit bar	Granose	360	102
Carob muesli/ pineapple bar	Granose	358	101
Carob fruit and nut	Allinson	543	154
ginger/bran biscuits		529	150
oatmeal biscuits		541	153
Carrots			
canned		19	5.5
old, boiled		19	5.5
old, raw		23	6.5
young, boiled		20	6
canned baby (sliced or whole)	Waitrose	18	5
canned drained	Tesco	18	5
canned sliced or whole	Hartley's	25	7
fresh, frozen, or canned and drained	Sainsbury	18	5
frozen	Ross	25	7
frozen baby	Birds Eye	18	5

Product	Brand	Calories per 100g/ 100ml	Calories per oz/ pack/ portion
Carrots and peas, fresh, frozen or canned and drained	Sainsbury	53	1tbsp/1oz 15
Cascade lemonade	Schweppes	20	6
Cashew nuts	St Michael	572	162
	Whitworths	530	150
roasted	Tesco	600	170
salted	Sainsbury	564	160
	Sun-Pat	585	166
Casilan (as sold)	Farley	376	107
Casserole Mix (Colman's) *see under flavours*			
Casserole vegetables	Birds Eye	35	10
	Ross	25	7
Castle marmalade	Baxters	253	12oz/340g jar 860
Castus fruit bars:	Granose		
apricot and date		244	69
date		268	76
date and coconut		280	79
date and nut		274	78
date and sesame		360	102
fig and date		224	64
Caterburgers	Ross	240	68
Catherine wheels	St Michael	310	88
Cauliflower			
boiled		*9*	*2.5*
raw		*13*	*4*
Cauliflower, fresh or frozen	Sainsbury	35	1 sprig/1oz 10
frozen	Birds Eye	18	5
	Waitrose	25	7

Product	Brand	Calories per 100g/ 100ml	Calories per oz/ pack/ portion
Cauliflower, peas and carrots	Birds Eye	35	10
Cauliflower, stir fry	St Michael	45	13
Cauliflower and cheese sauce	Birds Eye		per pack 290
Cauliflower cheese		*113*	*32*
Cauliflower cheese	St Michael	149	42
Cauliflower florets, frozen	Ross	25	7
	Tesco	25	7
Celeriac, boiled		*14*	*4*
Celery, boiled		*5*	*1.5*
raw		*8*	*2.5*
Celery, fresh, frozen, or canned and drained	Sainsbury		1 stick/ 1oz negl.
Celery salt	Tesco	100	28
Celery soup *see also Cream of celery*			
Celery soup (canned)	Sainsbury	53	½ pint 150
(dried)	Batchelors Cup-a-Soup	452	per portion 104
Cervelat	BHS	430	122
	Sainsbury	423	120
Champagne rhubarb yogurt	BHS	80	150g pack 121
Chapatis, made with fat		*336*	*95*
made without fat		*202*	*57*
CHEDDAR CHEESE	Prewetts	406	115
	Sainsbury	388	110
	Tesco	406	115
Canadian matured	Waitrose	423	120

Product	Brand	Calories per 100g/ 100ml	Calories per oz/ pack/ portion
CHEDDAR CHEESE			
Danish (50% fat in dry matter)	Danish	397	113
English or English matured	Waitrose	423	120
Irish	Waitrose	423	120
Irish white or red mature English	St Michael Cracker Barrel	405	115
		423	120
matured red, wedge or white	St Michael	403	114
mild – onion with chives	St Michael	372	105
mild – red	St Michael	400	113
mild – walnuts	St Michael	417	118
mild – white	St Michael	403	114
New Zealand	Waitrose	423	120
Scottish matured	Waitrose	423	120
traditional English matured	Waitrose	423	120
with walnuts	Sainsbury	423	120
Cheddar cheese spread, Canadian	Waitrose	374	106
Cheddar Cheshire cheese, white	Waitrose	388	110
Cheddar slices	Kraft	346	98
Cheddar spread	Kraft	296	84
	Primula	282	80
	Rowntree Mackintosh	285	81
Cheddars	Crawford		per biscuit 22

Product	Brand	Calories per 100g/100ml	Calories per oz/pack/portion
Cheese *see Camembert, etc, for branded packs*			
CHEESE			
Camembert type		300	85
Cheddar type		406	115
cottage		96	27
cream		439	124
Danish blue type		355	101
Edam type		304	86
Parmesan		408	116
processed		311	88
Cheese, bacon and onion flan	St Michael	298	84
Cheese, egg and bacon flan, large or small frozen	St Michael	261	74
	Birds Eye	325	5oz flan 460
		272	11oz flan 850
	BHS	280	79
Cheese, egg and onion flan	Birds Eye	325	5oz flan 460
		272	11oz flan 850
Cheese, onion and tomato pizza (100g)	Tiffany's	216	per pizza 216
Cheese and ham pancakes	Birds Eye		each, shallow fried 160
Cheese and ham pie (5oz)	Kraft Cheese Fayre	285	per pie 405
Cheese and onion crisps	BHS	530	150
	Safeway	559	158
	Sainsbury	540	25g 135
	St Michael	543	154

Product	Brand	Calories per 100g/ 100ml	Calories per oz/ pack/ portion
Cheese and onion crisps	Tesco	536	152
	Waitrose	550	156
Cheese and onion croquettes sizzle	Tiffany's	238	per croquette 124
Cheese and onion flan	St Michael	249	71
Cheese and onion fries	Ross	140	40
Cheese and onion hoops	BHS	505	143
Cheese and onion pasty (100g)	Kraft Cheese Fayre	295	84
Cheese and onion pie (142g/5oz)	Kraft Cheese Fayre	278	per pie 395
(5oz round, baked)	Tiffany's	280	per pie 397
Cheese and onion pizza (5in)	Ross	230	65
Cheese and onion puffs	Tesco	511	145
Cheese and onion savoury mash	Yeoman	386	per portion made up 72
Cheese and tomato pie (142g/oz)	Kraft Cheese Fayre	267	per pie 380
Cheese and tomato pizza	St Michael	239	68
7in	Ross	240	68
9in	Ross	220	62
100g	Tiffany's	223	63

Product	Brand	Calories per 100g/ 100ml	Calories per oz/ pack/ portion
Cheese and tomato Pot Noodle	Golden Wonder		carton made up 347
Cheese Crackles	BHS	533	151
Cheese Extra Specials	Crawford		per biscuit 53
Cheese flavoured potato snacks	Sainsbury	540	25g 135
Cheese flavoured puffs	Sainsbury	600	25g 150
Cheese pudding		*170*	*48*
Cheese puffs	BHS	550	156
	Tesco	541	153
Cheese sandwich biscuits	Sainsbury		per biscuit 35
	St Michael	520	per biscuit 52
	Tesco	511	145
Cheese sauce		*198*	*56*
Cheese sauce mix as sold	Colman's	415	118
	Knorr	429	122
made up	Chef Box	83	24
	Sainsbury	53	15
Cheese Savors	Crawford		per biscuit 3
Cheese savouries	Sainsbury		per biscuit 4
	Tesco	522	148
Cheese shapes	BHS	528	150
Cheese Snaps	St Michael	529	per biscuit 3
Cheese soufflé		*252*	*71*
Cheese spread		*283*	*80*
Cheese spread	Primula	282	80
	Safeway	290	82
	Sainsbury	247	1 tbsp/½oz 35

52

Product	Brand	Calories per 100g/ 100ml	Calories per oz/ pack/ portion
Cheese spread	Tesco	265	75
	Waitrose	290	82
(lactic cheese)	St Ivel	300	85
	Rowntree		
dairy	Mackintosh	260	74
with blue cheese	Primula	282	80
with celery	Primula	269	76
with chives	Primula	269	76
with crab	Primula	269	76
with ham	Kraft	275	78
	Primula	269	76
with ham and onion	Primula	269	76
with hot mixed peppers	Kraft	272	77
with onion	Kraft	289	82
	Primula	269	76
with pineapple	Primula	269	76
with shrimp	Kraft	282	80
	Primula	269	76
Cheese sticks	Sainsbury	500	25g 125
Cheese thins	BHS	535	152
	Sainsbury		per biscuit 20
Cheeseburger	Kraft Cheese Fayre		per burger well grilled 105
Cheesecake *see also Cherry, etc*			
Cheesecake		*421*	*119*
Cheesecake	Eden Vale	239	68
	Sainsbury	326	1/4 cake/2oz 185
fruit	Birds Eye		1/6 cake 260

53

Product	Brand	Calories per 100g/ 100ml	Calories per oz/ pack/ portion
Cheesecake mix	Safeway	394	141 crumb
		210	60 filling
plain (as sold)	Whitworths	510	7oz pack 1004
Cheeselets	Peek Frean	344	per biscuit 3.3
Cheesies	Birds Eye		each, grilled 75, fried 85
Chekwate drinks *see under flavours*			
Cherries, cooking			
raw		46	13
raw (with stones)		39	11
stewed with sugar		77	22
stewed with sugar (with stones)		67	19
stewed without sugar		39	11
stewed without sugar (with stones)		33	9.5
Cherries, eating			
raw		47	13
raw (with stones)		41	12
Cherries, fresh or frozen	Sainsbury	53	1 tbsp/1oz 15
Cherries, glacé *see Glacé*			
Cherry Bakewell tarts	BHS	425	per tart 207
Cherry brandy		255	72
Cherry butter sponge pudding	Tiffany's	160	¼ pudding 130
Cherry cake (round)	Tesco	438	124
Cherry cheesecake	St Michael	258	73
Cherry cheesecake mix (as sold)	Whitworths	430	11oz pack 1339

54

Product	Brand	Calories per 100g/ 100ml	Calories per oz/ pack/ portion
Cherry cocktail (canned, drained)	Tesco	203	58
Cherry cut cake	St Michael	394	112
Cherry dessert topping	Colman's	280	79
Cherry flan filling	Armour	115	33
Cherry Genoa cake	Waitrose	332	94
decorated square	St Michael	334	95
fully iced	St Michael	328	93
cut cake, all butter	St Michael	327	93
Cherry pie filling	Pack-a-Pie	66	per pack 269
	Sainsbury	141	1 tbsp/2oz 80
	Tesco	124	35
	Waitrose	99	28
Cherryade	Idris	25	7
	Tesco	23	6.5
sparkling	Corona	25	7
Cheshire cheese	Prewetts	382	108
	Sainsbury	317	90
red or white	St Michael	385	109
	Tesco	353	100
Cheshire slices	Kraft	342	97
Chestnuts (weighed with shells)		170	48
		140	40
Chewing nuts	Goodies	448	127
Chewits (all flavours)		381	108
Chewy fruits	Tesco	375	106
Chewy mints	Sainsbury	388	110
Chick peas (Bengal gram), raw		320	91
channa dahl		97	27
cooked, dahl		144	41

Product	Brand	Calories per 100g/100ml	Calories per oz/pack/portion
CHICKEN	British Poultry		
	Federation	190	54
	Waitrose	116	33
battercrisp thighs and drumsticks	St Michael	242	69
boiled			
dark meat		*204*	*58*
light meat		*163*	*46*
meat only (no skin)		*183*	*52*
breast fillets	St Michael	114	32
breasts	St Michael	186	53
crumbed breast fillets, thighs, etc	St Michael	289	82
drumsticks	St Michael	162	46
leg quarter (with bone)		*92*	*26*
liver *see Liver*			
raw			
dark meat		*126*	*36*
light meat		*116*	*33*
meat and skin		*230*	*65*
meat only		*121*	*34*
roast			
dark meat		*155*	*44*
light meat		*142*	*40*
meat and skin		*216*	*61*
meat only		*148*	*42*
roast			
joint	Sainsbury	82	6oz joint 140
slices	Sainsbury	141	1 slice/1oz 40
whole or portions	St Michael	216	61

Product	Brand	Calories per 100g/ 100ml	Calories per oz/ pack/ portion
CHICKEN			
roast breast of (sliced meat)	St Michael	210	60
spring	St Michael	213	60
stuffed breasts	St Michael	197	56
stuffed thighs	St Michael	211	60
Tandoori	St Michael	240	68
thighs	St Michael	237	67
whole fresh	St Michael	213	60
whole leg	St Michael	237	67
wing quarter (weighed with bone)		74	*21*
wings	St Michael	126	36
Chicken and asparagus pie (1½lb), baked	Tiffany's	250	¼ pie 450
Chicken and bacon spread	Country Pot	155	44
Chicken and celery soup, low calorie	Waistline	11	3
Chicken and ham paste	Princes	200	57
	Shippams	200	57
Chicken and ham pie	BHS	264	large pie 1200
		228	small pie 387
	Kraft	317	per 340g/12 oz pie 1080
	Safeway	300	86
frozen	Safeway	300	86
	Sainsbury	282	¼ pie/3¾oz 300
Chicken and herbs Pasta Menu	Crosse & Blackwell	95	27

57

Product	Brand	Calories per 100g/ 100ml	Calories per oz/ pack/ portion
Chicken and leek soup, dried as sold	Cup-a-Soup	414	per portion 91
	Knorr	338	96
made up	Chef Box	27	7.5
	Sainsbury	42	½ pint 120
Chicken and mushroom casserole	Birds Eye		per pack 160
Chicken and mushroom Omelette Mate	Campbell's	54	15
Chicken and mushroom pancakes (shallow fried)	Birds Eye		per pancake 150
Chicken and mushroom pie	Birds Eye		indiv. pie 350
	BHS	243	149g pie 362
	Fray Bentos	212	60 142g/5oz pie 305
baked	Tiffany's	245	5oz round pie 345
small	St Michael	282	80
Chicken and mushroom pie filling	Fray Bentos	95	26
Chicken and mushroom Pot Noodle	Golden Wonder		carton made up 381
Chicken and mushroom soup	Batchelors 5-Minute		per pack 219
Chicken and mushroom Toast Topper	Heinz	74	21
Chicken and vegetable broth with rice (undiluted)	Granny's	36	10

Product	Brand	Calories per 100g/ 100ml	Calories per oz/ pack/ portion
Chicken and vegetable pie			
4½oz oval, baked	Tiffany's	250	per pie 320
5oz round, baked	Tiffany's	235	per pie 333
1lb, baked	Tiffany's	245	¼ pie 275
fresh	Tesco	236	67
Chicken and vegetable soup	Heinz Big Soups	48	14
undiluted	Campbell's Main-Course	59	17
low calorie	Heinz	21	6
Chicken broth	Baxters	33	15oz/425g can 141
	Heinz Big Soups	66	19
thick (as sold)	Knorr	345	98
Chicken casserole ready meal	Ross	70	20
Chicken chasseur (Cook in the Pot)	Crosse & Blackwell	389	110
Chicken chasseur Casserole Mix (as sold)	Colman's	245	69
Chicken croquettes, sizzle (as sold)	Tiffany's	260	per croquette 150
Chicken curry, canned	Tesco	155	44
Chicken curry Pot Rice	Golden Wonder		carton made up 264
Chicken curry with rice frozen	Birds Eye		per pack 400
	BHS	94	per 228g pack 214

59

Product	Brand	Calories per 100g/ 100ml	Calories per oz/ pack/ portion
Chicken curry with separate rice	Crosse & Blackwell	96	27
Chicken drumsticks, fried	Ross	210	60
Chicken flavour crisps	BHS	530	150
Chicken in jelly	St Michael	180	51
Chicken in the basket	St Michael	441	125
Chicken in white sauce	Sainsbury	164	7oz can 325
	Tesco	250	71
Chicken kebabs	St Michael	153	43
Chicken Kiev	St Michael	322	91
Chicken liver pâté	Princes	336	95
Chicken noodle soup, condensed (undiluted)	Campbell's	39	11
Chicken noodle soup, dried		329	93
(as served)		20	6
Chicken noodle soup, dried (as sold)	Knorr	338	96
	Tesco	368	104
dried (made up)	Chef Box Maggi Quick	26	7.5
	Cook	26	7.5
	Sainsbury	14	½ pint 40
Chicken paste (78g)	Shippams	220	62
Chicken pie	Birds Eye		indiv. pie 410 pie for 2–3 1080

Product	Brand	Calories per 100g/ 100ml	Calories per oz/ pack/ portion
Chicken pie	Brains		family pie 1095
	Kraft	340	113g/4oz pie 385
canned	Tesco	212	60
family	Ross	260	74
frozen	Tesco	286	81
individual	Ross	290	82
Chicken portions (cooked, meat only)	Ross	240	68
Chicken rice soup, condensed (undiluted)	Campbell's	53	15
Chicken rissoles (as sold)	Tiffany's	260	per rissole 130
Chicken roll	BHS	140	113g pack 159
Chicken seasoning (as sold)	Colman's	360	102
Chicken soup *see also Cream of chicken*			
Chicken soup	BHS	57	16
canned	Sainsbury	60	½ pint 170
condensed (undiluted)	Campbell's Bumper Harvest	52	15
	Granny's	64	18
dried (as sold)	Batchelors		per portion
	Cup-a-Soup	433	104
	Knorr Quick	413	117
dried (made up)	Sainsbury	42	½ pint 120
low calorie	Heinz	23	6.5
	Slim-a-Soup		11g portion 36

Product	Brand	Calories per 100g/ 100ml	Calories per oz/ pack/ portion
Chicken soup			
supreme	Sainsbury	74	½ pint 210
thick			
(dried, made up)	Chef Box Maggi	30	8.5
	Quick Cook	30	8.5
Chicken Spread	Shippams	190	54
Chicken spread with mushroom	Country Pot	155	44
Chicken stew	Campbell's	69	20
Chicken stock *see also* **Oxo**			
(undiluted)	Campbell's	75	21
cubes	Fray Bentos	300	85
	Knorr	304	86
powder	Knorr	173	49
tablets	Safeway	326	93
Chicken supreme	Birds Eye		per pack 250
	Crosse & Blackwell	128	36
	Snackpot	382	per pot 241
	Vesta	369	per pack 813
Today's Special (undiluted)	Campbell's	123	35
Chicklets	Birds Eye		each, grilled 160, fried 195
Chicory, raw		9	2.5
Chicory beverage	Prewetts	256	73
Chili con Carne	Goblin	151	297g pack 450
	Vesta	360	per pack 803
Cook in the Pot	Crosse & Blackwell	382	108

62

Product	Brand	Calories per 100g/ 100ml	Calories per oz/ pack/ portion
Chilli con Carne Casserole Mix (as sold)	Colman's	295	84
Chilli Cook-in-Sauce	Homepride	104	376g pack 390
Chipolatas			
beef	Tesco	320	91
	Waitrose	289	82
pork	Tesco	358	101
pork and beef	Tesco	328	93
Chips		*253*	*72*
CHIPS			
crinkle cut	BHS	296	2lb pack 2688
	Ross	140	40
	St Michael	109	31
	Tesco	198	56
deep fried	Birds Eye	247	70
shallow fried	Birds Eye	229	65
fresh or frozen, fried	Sainsbury	229	65
frozen		*109*	*31*
fried		*291*	*82*
frozen	Safeway	239	68
	Waitrose	240	68
Jacket	Ross	120	35
Just Bake	St Michael	208	59
oven	BHS	90	2lb pack 815
	Ross	150	42
	Tesco	150	42
baked or grilled	Birds Eye	194	55

Product	Brand	Calories per 100g/ 100ml	Calories per oz/ pack/ portion
CHIPS			
steak (as sold)	Ross	110	30
straight cut	BHS	231	2lb pack 2100
	Ross	120	35
	Tesco	198	56
deep fried	Birds Eye	247	70
shallow fried	Birds Eye	229	65
Chive mustard	Colman's	170	48
Choc and nut capri Italiano (585g/1 litre)	Wall's	197	per pack 1155
Choc and nut slice (282g)	Wall's	186	per pack 525
Choc bar	Wall's		
Dark and Golden			each 130
Double Choc			each 160
Golden Vanilla			each 130
Midnight Mint			each 140
Choc chip cookies	Tesco	484	137
Choc chip 'n' nut cookies	Huntley & Palmers	476	per biscuit 44
Choc ice *see also Cornish, etc.*			
Choc ice (pack of 6)	Tesco	150	43
Choc mint	Lyons Maid		each 168
Choc 'n' nut cookies	BHS	500	142
Choc 'n' nut supermousse	Birds Eye		per tub 150
Choc-a-Block	BHS	471	134
Choc-o-lait	Crawford		per biscuit 58
Chocolate *see also Milk, Plain, etc.*			

Product	Brand	Calories per 100g/ 100ml	Calories per oz/ pack/ portion
CHOCOLATE			
fancy and filled		460	130
milk		529	150
milk	Sainsbury	582	165
milk, Ovaltine	Wander	505	50g pack 36 100g pack 31
plain		525	149
plain	Sainsbury	546	155
Swiss milk	St Michael	533	151
soft filled	St Michael	614	174
Swiss plain	St Michael	524	149
Chocolate and cherry gâteau	St Michael	272	77
Chocolate and mint mousse	Tesco	163	46
Chocolate and nut cookies	Sainsbury		per biscuit 45
Chocolate and orange cookies	St Michael	476	per biscuit 79
Chocolate Assortment	Waitrose	469	133
Chocolate biscuit fingers	McVitie		per biscuit 27
Chocolate biscuits *see also Milk, Plain*			
Chocolate biscuits, full-coated		524	149
Chocolate blancmange (as sold)	Brown & Polson	331	35g pack 116
Chocolate buttercream roll	Sainsbury	353	1/6 roll/ 1½oz 150
Chocolate Buttons	Cadbury's	523	148
milk	Sainsbury	494	140

Product	Brand	Calories per 100g/ 100ml	Calories per oz/ pack/ portion
Chocolate cake	Sainsbury	423	⅕ cake/ 2oz 240
	Waitrose	497	141
Chocolate Caprice	Lyons	460	per cake 140
Chocolate chip cookies	St Michael	494	per biscuit 52
Chocolate chip ice cream	St Michael	263	75
Chocolate coated roll	Tesco	418	119
Chocolate coffee beans	BHS	490	139
Chocolate covered mini rolls	Sainsbury		per roll 145
Chocolate covered Swiss roll small	Waitrose	437	124
	Waitrose	363	103
Chocolate covered buttercream Swiss roll (small)	Waitrose	444	126
Chocolate Cream	Fry's	414	117
Chocolate cream biscuits	Sainsbury		per biscuit 65
Chocolate cream dessert	Eden Vale	143	41
Chocolate cup cakes	Lyons	318	per cake 129
	Sainsbury		per cake 130
	Waitrose	688	195
Chocolate Delight made up	St Michael	139	39
	Tesco	155	44

Product	Brand	Calories per 100g/ 100ml	Calories per oz/ pack/ portion
Chocolate dessert	BHS	99	105g pack 104
	Sainsbury		per tub 210
	St Michael	144	41
	Waitrose	452	128
Chocolate dessert sauce	HP Foods	305	86
	Lyons Maid	283	80
	Tesco	331	94
	Wall's	114	250g pack 285
Chocolate dessert topping	Colman's	300	85
Chocolate digestive biscuits *see also Digestive*			
Chocolate digestive biscuits		*493*	*140*
Chocolate éclairs (cakes, 5 per pack)	St Michael	413	per éclair 127
Chocolate éclairs (sweets)	Tesco	437	124
Chocolate éclairs, Cadbury (sweets)	Pascall	441	125
Chocolate filled roll	Tesco	409	116
Chocolate filled wafers	Sainsbury		per biscuit 30
Chocolate flavour drink	Cup-a-Time	370	per pack 118
Chocolate flavoured candy products	Goodies	532	151
Chocolate flavoured milk drink	St Michael	101	29
Chocolate flavoured roll	Sainsbury	338	$1/7$ large or $1/5$ small/1oz 110
Chocolate fool	Eden Vale	217	62

Product	Brand	Calories per 100g/ 100ml	Calories per oz/ pack/ portion
Chocolate fresh cream dessert	St Ivel	154	44
Chocolate fudge cake	BHS	355	303g cake 1077
Chocolate gâteau	Birds Eye		1/6 cake 200
	Tesco	456	129
Chocolate ice cream	Lyons Maid	family brick 401	
	Sainsbury	176	1/5 block/ 2fl.oz 50
	Tudor	180	51
Chocolate iced tarts	Lyons	395	per tart 119
Chocolate instant dessert (made up)	Safeway	137	39
Chocolate Jelly Cream (as sold)	Chivers	365	103
Chocolate junior rolls with choc.	Sainsbury		per roll 120
buttercream	St Michael	465	per roll 133
Chocolate layer gâteau	St Michael	340	96
Chocolate limes	Parkinsons	404	114
Chocolate lolly (multipack)	Lyons Maid		each 46
Chocolate Lovely	Birds Eye		per tub 220
Chocolate malted milk biscuits	Sainsbury		per biscuit 45
Chocolate mint leaves	BHS	474	134
Chocolate mint sundaes	BHS	535	152

Product	Brand	Calories per 100g/ 100ml	Calories per oz/ pack/ portion
Chocolate mousse	Birds Eye		per tub 110
	Tesco	165	47
	Waitrose	102	29
Wizard	St Ivel	175	50
Chocolate nougat	BHS	416	50g pack 208
Chocolate nut meringue	St Michael	299	85
Chocolate Oliver biscuits	Fortts	389	per biscuit 21
Chocolate orange slices	BHS	474	134
Chocolate peanuts	Tesco	540	153
Chocolate peanuts and raisins	Tesco	480	136
Chocolate peppermint creams	Sainsbury	388	110
Chocolate ripple cutting brick	Tudor Lyons Maid	180	51 per pack 925
Chocolate roll	BHS	426	210g roll 895
Chocolate rum flavour truffles	BHS	415	118
Chocolate sandwich cake	BHS	490	298g cake 1459
	Sainsbury	353	1/5 cake/1½oz 150
Chocolate sandwich wafers	Sainsbury		per wafer 90
Chocolate sauce	St Michael	255	72
Chocolate soufflé	St Ivel	185	52

Product	Brand	Calories per 100g/ 100ml	Calories per oz/ pack/ portion
Chocolate sponge cake mix (as sold)	Whitworths	352	6½oz pack 649
fully made up	Sainsbury	413	¹/₆ cake/3½oz 410
Chocolate sponge pudding	Goblin	240	297g pudding 715
	Heinz	316	90
	St Michael	373	106
Chocolate sponge roll	Lyons	400	per roll 1016
	St Michael	408	116
Chocolate sponge sandwich	Lyons	373	per cake 858
with vanilla	Tiffany's	468	¼ cake 234
Chocolate sponge sandwich mix	Sainsbury	380	¹/₁₆ cake/2½oz 270 made up
Chocolate sponge slice	Lyons	362	per cake 681
Chocolate Sports	McVitie		each 114
Chocolate spread	Cadbury's	320	91
	Sainsbury	317	1 tbsp/½oz 45
Chocolate stem ginger	BHS	597	169
Chocolate Supermousse	Birds Eye		per tub 120
Chocolate supreme dessert	Sainsbury		pkt made up 485
Chocolate Swiss roll	BHS	402	182g roll 732
	Lyons	359	per roll 632
	St Michael	397	113
	Waitrose	395	112

Product	Brand	Calories per 100g/ 100ml	Calories per oz/ pack/ portion
Chocolate toffee rolls	Callard & Bowser, Nuttall	460	per sweet 34
	Tesco	452	128
Chocolate toffees box, bag or loose	Callard & Bowser, Nuttall	460	per sweet 39
roll	Callard & Bowser, Nuttall	460	per sweet 22
Chocolate Two Shakes	Kellogg's	366 (100g dry)	½ sachet (20g) + ½ pint milk 274
Chocolate teacakes	Sainsbury		per biscuit 70
Chocolate vanilla Swiss roll	Waitrose	388	110
Chocolate Vienna	McVitie		per biscuit 50
Chocolate whip	St Michael	185	52
Chocolate wholemeal milk	Crawford		per biscuit 78
plain	Crawford		per biscuit 77
Chocolate yogurt	Eden Vale	96	27
	Sainsbury	127	sm. tub/ ¼ pint 180
Choice celery soup	Batchelors 5-Minute		per pack 188
Chop Sauce	Tesco	81	23
Chop Suey	Vesta	341	per pack 873
Chop Suey (as sold)	Breakfast	270	per pack 310

Product	Brand	Calories per 100g/ 100ml	Calories per oz/ pack/ portion
Chopped beef grill (frozen)	Sainsbury	229	65
Chopped ham and pork (canned)		270	77
Chopped ham and pork (canned)	Libby	270	77
Chopped ham and pork (canned)	Tesco	339	96
Chopped ham loaf (canned)	Sainsbury	247	1 thin slice/ 1oz 70
Chopped ham roll	Sainsbury		1 slice 50
Chopped ham with pork	Armour	330	94
Chopped pork and ham (canned or sliced)	Waitrose	342	97
Chopped veal steaks	Ross	240	68
Chorley cakes (4 per pack)	St Michael	408	per cake 290
Choux buns			
(2 per pack)	St Michael	330	per bun 257
(4 per pack)	Birds Eye		per bun 125
Chow Mein	Vesta	279	per pack 466
Christmas (Xmas) cake, fully iced luxury iced top all butter	St Michael	319	90
madeira	St Michael	413	117
Christmas pudding		304	86
Christmas pudding	Crosse & Blackwell	321	91
	Robertson's	296	84
	Safeway	325	92
	St Michael	354	100

Product	Brand	Calories per 100g/ 100ml	Calories per oz/ pack/ portion
Chunky chicken (canned)	St Michael	150	43
Chunky chicken in barbecue sauce	Shippams	135	38
in curry sauce	Shippams	120	34
in mushroom sauce	Shippams	150	43
in savoury white sauce	Shippams	150	43
Chunky salad	St Michael	14	4
Chunky steak (canned)	St Michael	176	50
Chutney			
apple		*193*	*55*
tomato		*154*	*44*
Cider *see also under brand names*			
Cider, dry		*36*	*10*
sweet		*42*	*12*
vintage		*101*	*29*
Cinnamon, ground	Tesco	250	71
	Whitworths	232	66
Clear fruits	Pascall	376	107
	Sainsbury	335	95
Clear mints	Sainsbury	335	95
Cloves, whole	Tesco	400	113
Club biscuits:	Jacobs		
fruit		478	each 111
milk		502	each 114
mint		495	each 113
orange		497	each 113
plain		494	each 112
wafer		516	each 97

Product	Brand	Calories per 100g/ 100ml	Calories per oz/ pack/ portion
Clubsteak (as sold)	Tiffany's	250	3oz steak 170
Coasters	Cadbury's	488	138
Coat & Cook *see under flavours*			
Cob or hazel nuts (weighed with shells)		380	108
		137	39
Coburg bread	St Michael	250	71
Coca-cola		39	11
Coca Cola	Coca Cola	43	185ml 80, 325ml 140
Cock-a-Leekie soup	Baxters	14	15oz can 60
	BHS	14	per can 60
Cockles, boiled		48	14
Cocktail onions	Crosse & Blackwell	2	
Coco Krispies	Kellogg's	355	101
Cocoa (made up)	Sainsbury	77	½ pint (3tsp + half milk/ water) 220
Cocoa powder		312	88
Cocoa powder	Rowntree Mackintosh	350	99
Coconut, desiccated		604	171
Coconut, desiccated	Safeway	627	178
	Tesco	604	171
	Whitworths	604	171
fresh		351	100
Coconut biscuits	Allinson	564	160
Coconut cake	St Michael	415	118
Coconut cakes	BHS	440	125

Product	Brand	Calories per 100g/ 100ml	Calories per oz/ pack/ portion
Coconut cookies	Sainsbury		per biscuit 45
	Waitrose	497	141
Coconut cream biscuits	Waitrose	511	145
Coconut crumble creams	Tesco	524	149
Coconut crunch cake	BHS	586	166
Coconut crunch cakes	Sainsbury		per cake 150
Coconut crunch cookies	BHS	490	139
Coconut crunchies	Sainsbury		per biscuit 45
Coconut cup cakes	Sainsbury		per cake 115
Coconut flake	Lyons Maid		each 172
Coconut macaroons	Tesco	476	135
Coconut mallows	Peek Frean	384	per biscuit 46
Coconut milk		*21*	*6*
Coconut mushrooms	St Michael	432	122
Coconut rings (plain)	Tesco	483	137
Chocolate	Tesco	471	134
COD			
baked		*96*	*27*
(with bones and skin)		*82*	*23*
breaded fillets (frozen)	BHS	150	43
chunky (frozen)	BHS		per pack 212
Crispy (battered, as sold)	Ross	170	48
crispy, and chips	Birds Eye		per pack, fried 540
dried salt, boiled		*138*	*39*

Product	Brand	Calories per 100g/ 100ml	Calories per oz/ pack/ portion
COD			
Faroese fillets (fresh)	St Michael	74	21
fillet (frozen)	Birds Eye	71	20
fillets (fresh, raw)		*76*	*22*
fillets (frozen)	BHS	80	23
	Ross	80	23
	Waitrose	81	23
fried	Waitrose	141	40
Fillets in breadcrumbs	Ross	120	34
	St Michael	118	33
Fillets (smoked)	St Michael	82	23
fillets and steaks (fresh or frozen)	Sainsbury	70	20
fried (frozen)	Waitrose	141	40
fried in batter		*199*	*56*
grilled		*95*	*27*
oven (battered, as sold)	Ross	200	57
poached		*94*	*27*
(with bones and skin)		*82*	*23*
shop fried (frozen)	Safeway	140	40
skinless fillets (as sold)	Ross	80	23
skinless boneless fillets (fresh)	St Michael	74	21
smoked (fresh or frozen)	Sainsbury	70	20
poached		*101*	*29*
raw		*79*	*22*

Product	Brand	Calories per 100g/ 100ml	Calories per oz/ pack/ portion
COD			
steaks, frozen		*68*	*19*
steamed		*83*	*24*
(frozen)	Safeway	*82*	*23*
(with bones and skin)		*67*	*19*
Cod and prawn pie	St Michael	165	47
Cod bake (as sold)	Ross	120	34
Cod crumble (as sold)	Ross	180	51
Cod fingers, crispy	Birds Eye		per finger, fried 65
Cod fingers, Jumbo (as sold)	Ross	170	48
Cod fish fingers	Birds Eye		per finger, fried 65, grilled 55
	St Michael	168	48
Cod fries, crispy	Birds Eye	176	per pack, deep fried 390, shallow fried 430
Cod in batter, fried	Sainsbury	212	60
Cod in breadcrumbs (frozen)	Tesco	107	30
Cod in breadcrumbs, grilled or fried (with a little oil)	Sainsbury	212	60
Cod in butter sauce	Birds Eye		per pack 195
	BHS	90	per pack 135
	Sainsbury	94	6oz pack 160
Cod with butter sauce	Tesco	73	21

Product	Brand	Calories per 100g/ 100ml	Calories per oz/ pack/ portion
Cod in cheese sauce	Birds Eye		per pack 195
Cod in mushroom sauce	Birds Eye		per pack 190
Cod in parsley sauce	Birds Eye		per pack 175
	St Michael	94	27
Cod with parsley sauce	Tesco	68	19
Cod in shrimp flavour sauce	Birds Eye		per pack 180
Cod liver oil		899	255
Cod pie, chunky (as sold)	Ross	150	43
Cod portions, crispy	Birds Eye		per portion, fried 140
Cod portions	Sainsbury	70	20
Cod Provençale	BHS	90	26
Cod roe, hard			
fried		202	57
raw		113	32
Cod roes, pressed	John West	104	29
Cod steaks	Birds Eye		per steak 80
as sold	Ross	80	23
crispy	Birds Eye		per steak, deep fried 215, shallow fried 190
oven crispy	Birds Eye		per steak, baked or grilled 215
in batter	Tesco	200	57

Product	Brand	Calories per 100g/ 100ml	Calories per oz/ pack/ portion
Cod steaks			
in breadcrumbs (as sold)	Ross	120	34
in butter sauce	Ross	80	23
in crisp crunch crumb	Birds Eye		per steak, grilled or baked 185, shallow fried 210
in parsley sauce (as sold)	Ross	60	17
Coffee, Continental			
granules (dry)	Waitrose	88	25
extra flavour (dry)	Waitrose	88	25
freeze dried (made up)	Safeway	negl.	negl.
ground, roasted (dry)		*287*	*81*
ground (dry)	Waitrose	300	85
ground fresh (made up)	Safeway	negl.	negl.
infusion (5 minutes)		*2*	
instant (dry)		*100*	*28*
instant (dry)	Tesco	105	30
	Waitrose	88	25
instant (made up)	Safeway	negl.	negl.
Coffee and chicory essence		*218*	*62*
Coffee chocolates	Callard & Bowser, Nuttall	420	per sweet 29

Product	Brand	Calories per 100g/ 100ml	Calories per oz/ pack/ portion
Coffee Compliment	Cadbury's	536	152
Coffee creams	Peek Frean	476	per biscuit 57
	Tesco	459	130
Coffee ice cream	Sainsbury	194 (100g)	¹/₅ block/ 2fl.oz 55
Coffee mandarin gâteau	Ross	300	85
Coffee roll	Sainsbury	376	¹/₆ roll/ 1½oz 160
Coffee sponge sandwich	Lyons	408	per cake 959
Coffee toffees	Callard & Bowser, Nuttall	470	per sweet 40
Coffee-Mate	Carnation	353	per rounded tsp. 10
Cognac liqueur bar	St Michael	467	132
Cola	Britvic	41	12
	Safeway	20–30	6–9
	Sainsbury	40	½ pint 115
	Slimsta	4	1
	Tesco	27	7.5
	Waitrose	40	12
(320ml)	BHS	45	per pack 143
(1½ litres)	BHS	26	7
canned	Safeway	43	12
Strike	Barr	32	9
Coleslaw	BHS	126	226g pack 285
	Eden Vale	126	36
	Heinz	127	36
	Sainsbury	141	1 tbsp/1oz 40

Product	Brand	Calories per 100g/ 100ml	Calories per oz/ pack/ portion
Coleslaw	St Ivel	120	34
	St Michael	172	49
	Tesco	126	36
coarse cut	Eden Vale	125	35
coarse cut, with			
pineapple	BHS	118	226g pack 267
Low Calorie	Tesco	48	14
low calorie (canned)	Tesco	53	15
prawn	BHS	108	200g pack 216
in low calorie			
dressing	St Ivel	60	17
in vinaigrette	BHS	33	9.5
	St Ivel	95	27
	Tesco	60	17
with cheese	Sainsbury	159	1 tbsp/1oz 45
with French			
mayonnaise	St Michael	340	96
with prawns	Sainsbury	141	1 tbsp/1oz 40
with vinaigrette	Sainsbury	70	1 tbsp/1oz 20
Coleslaw dressing	Kraft	462	131
Coley (frozen)	Safeway	70	20
fillet (fresh or frozen)	Sainsbury	70	20
Complan (powder):	Farley		57g sachet
butterscotch		436	248
chocolate		440	251
natural or strawberry		444	253
Compound cooking fat		894	253
Condensed milk, sweetened			
skimmed		267	76
whole		322	91

Product	Brand	Calories per 100g/ 100ml	Calories per oz/ pack/ portion
Condensed milk, sweetened	Fussell's Blue Butterfly	267	76
	Nestle	325	92
	Sainsbury		1 tbsp 90
Cones	Wall's		large 25 medium 10 sugar 40
Consommé	Frank Cooper	12	15oz can 52
	Crosse & Blackwell	22	6
(undiluted)	Campbell's	32	9
supreme	Sainsbury	21	½ pint 60
Continental stir-fry vegetables (fried)	Birds Eye	88	25
Contrast Assortment	Cadbury's	451	128
Cook-in-Sauces (Baxters) see under flavours			
Cook in the Pot (Crosse & Blackwell) see Madras Curry, etc			
Cookies	Cadbury's	485	137
Cooking fat	Van den Berghs	894	253
Cooking fat, compound		*894*	*253*
Cooking oil	Van den Berghs	899	255
Coola (bottled)	Idris	39	11
Coola sparkling drink	Corona	39	11
Coolmints	Trebor		per pack 90 per sweet 6.5
Coq au Vin Casserole Mix (as sold)	Colman's	245	69

Product	Brand	Calories per 100g/ 100ml	Calories per oz/ pack/ portion
Corn see also Corn on the cob, Sweetcorn			
Corn			
cream style	Green		
(canned)	Giant	85	24
niblets	Green		
(canned or frozen)	Giant	83	23
raw (frozen)	Safeway	96	28
Corn crisp	BHS	457	170g pack 777
	Sainsbury	423	1/s cake/1oz 120
	St Michael	457	per cake 130
	Waitrose	511	145
Corn curls	Tesco	170	48
Corn Flakes see also Cornflakes			
Corn Flakes	Kellogg's	344	98
Crunchy Nut	Kellogg's	372	105
Corn Oil	Mazola	900	255
	Safeway	900	255
	Tesco	932	264
	Waitrose	924	262
Corn on the cob			
boiled		123	35
raw		127	36
Corn on the cob	Birds Eye	70	7oz 140
Corn on the cob, frozen			8–9oz 170
			10oz–200
(2 ears or	Green		
4 half ears)	Giant	88	25
Corn relish	BHS	109	31
	Tesco	109	31
Corned beef, canned		217	62

Product	Brand	Calories per 100g/ 100ml	Calories per oz/ pack/ portion
Corned beef, canned	Armour	232	66
	Fray Bentos	215	61
	Libby	200	57
(Argentine or Scottish)	St Michael	217	62
sliced	St Michael	217	62
Corned beef hash savoury (as sold)	Tiffany's	200	per savoury 184
Corned beef salad	BHS	287	81
Cornetto:	Wall's		
choc and nut			per cone 195
mint choc chip			per cone 220
raspberry crush			per cone 175
rum and raisin			per cone 195
strawberry			per cone 185
Cornflakes		*368*	*104*
Cornflakes	Safeway	354	100
	Sainsbury	353	4tbsp/½oz 50
	Tesco	354	100
	Waitrose	367	104
Cornflour		*354*	*100*
Cornflour	Safeway	354	100
	Tesco	350	99
Patent	Brown & Polson	328	93
Cornish choc sundae	Lyons Maid		each 133
Cornish creams	Safeway	507	145
Cornish dairy ice cream	Lyons Maid		per cutting brick 903 per family brick 428

Product	Brand	Calories per 100g/ 100ml	Calories per oz/ pack/ portion
Cornish ice cream	Safeway	204	59
Cornish ice cream bar	Wall's		per bar 90
Cornish pastie		*332*	*94*
Cornish pasties	Ross	280	79
	Tesco	281	80
85g/3oz	Kraft	347	per pasty 295
100g	Tiffany's	245	per pasty 245
155g	BHS	452	per pasty 700
individual	Sainsbury		per pasty 480
large	Sainsbury	366	per pasty 1610
pack of 4	BHS		per pasty 300
pack of 4	St Michael	277	79
savoury	Sainsbury	317	90
single	St Michael	231	65
traditional	St Michael	340	96
Cornish raspberry sundae	Lyons Maid		each 97
Cornish style vegetables with chicken	Knorr Hot Pots	380	45g pack 175
Cornish vanilla choc ice	Lyons Maid		each 126
Cornish vanilla Kup	Lyons Maid		each 110
Cornish Wafers	Jacobs	527	per biscuit 44
	Tesco	549	156
Cottage cheese	Sainsbury	106	1 tbs/1oz 30
apple, nuts and sultana	St Michael	120	34
cheddar & onion	BHS	121	226g pack 273
	Eden Vale	121	34

Product	Brand	Calories per 100g/ 100ml	Calories per oz/ pack/ portion
Cottage cheese			
cheddar cheese and			
onion	St Michael	127	36
chive	Eden Vale	97	27
chives	St Michael	97	27
natural	BHS	97	226g pack 219
	Eden Vale	97	27
	St Ivel	100	28
onion and cheddar	St Ivel	118	33
onion & peppers	Eden Vale	86	24
pineapple	Eden Vale	86	24
	St Ivel	97	27
	St Michael	86	24
plain	St Michael	100	28
prawn	St Ivel	126	36
prawns	St Michael	130	37
salmon and			
cucumber	Eden Vale	116	33
	St Michael	116	33
vegetable and ham	St Ivel	105	30
with chives	BHS	97	226g pack 219
with pineapple	BHS	86	226g pack 195
Cottage pie	Brains		per pie 455
	BHS	165	399g pie 658
5oz round (baked)	Tiffany's	260	per pie 370
family	St Michael	147	42
fresh	Tesco	198	56
large	St Michael	130	37
small	St Michael	163	46
Cottage vegetable *soup, rich*	Batchelors 5-Minute		per pack 193

Product	Brand	Calories per 100g/ 100ml	Calories per oz/ pack/ portion
Counters	Mars		per sweet 6 per standard pack 147
Countess yogurt	St Ivel	117	33 (average)
Country bran	Jordans	293	83
Country bran bread	St Michael	236	67
Country cake	BHS	394	390g cake 1536
	St Michael	405	115
Country chicken and leek soup	Batchelors 5-Minute		per pack 181
Country chicken noodle soup	Batchelors 5-Minute		per pack 154
Country mix vegetables	Ross	40	11
Country muesli	Jordans	352	100
Country mushroom soup (as sold)	Knorr	384	109
Country mushroom soup, rich	Batchelors 5-Minute		per pack 211
Country pickle	Baxters	165	305g jar 503
Country Pots see under flavours			
Country Prize yogurt:	St Ivel		
grapefruit muesli		83	24
muesli		96	27
walnut muesli		88	25
Country salad	Eden Vale	125	35
Country stir-fry vegetables (fried)	Birds Eye	88	25

Product	Brand	Calories per 100g/ 100ml	Calories per oz/ pack/ portion
Country Store	Kellogg's	353	100
Country style cut cake	St Michael	360	102
Country style fruit cake	Waitrose	367	104
Country style pâté	St Michael	300	85
Country vegetable soup, thick (dried, as sold)	Knorr Hearty	332	94
thick (dried, made up)	Chef Box Maggi Quick Cook	32	9
		33	9.5
Country vegetable spread	Waistline	85	24
Country vegetable with beef soup	Crosse & Blackwell	41	12
Courgettes, fresh, frozen or canned and drained	Sainsbury	35	1tbsp/1oz 10
sliced	Birds Eye	14	4 (boiled)
		60	17 (fried)
Crab, boiled		*127*	*36*
boiled (with shell)		*25*	*7*
canned		*81*	*23*
Crab, dressed	John West	138	39
Crab bisque	Frank Cooper	47	15oz can 195
Crab paste (78g)	Shippams	160	45
Crab pâté (35g)	Shippams	155	44
Crab salad	BHS	394	112
Crab spread	Princes	146	41

Product	Brand	Calories per 100g/100ml	Calories per oz/pack/portion
Crabmeat	Armour	81	23
Cracked wheat bread	St Michael	222	63
Cranberries, raw		*15*	*4.5*
Cranberry jelly	Crosse & Blackwell	259	73
Cranberry sauce, jellied	Baxters	253	6oz/177g jar 574
whole fruit	Baxters	225	6oz/177g jar 510
Cranberry sauce and wine	Colman's	215	61
CREAM			
canned (sterilized)		*230*	*65*
canned (sterilized)	Fussell's Golden Butterfly	233	66
	Nestlé	233	66
	Safeway	233	66
	Tesco	243	69
clotted	St Ivel	575	163
Cornish	St Michael	574	163
	Tesco	560	159
Devon	Tesco	590	167
double		*447*	*127*
double	BHS	440	114ml 502 228ml 1003
	Eden Vale	450	128
	Safeway	460	131
	Sainsbury		1 tbsp 85
	St Ivel	450	128

Product	Brand	Calories per 100g/100ml	Calories per oz/pack/portion
CREAM, *double*	St Michael	450	128
	Tesco	448	127
	Waitrose	462	131
extra-thick	Tesco	290	82
extra-thick double	Waitrose	462	131
extra-thick texture	BHS	290	82
extra-thick with rum	Tesco	430	122
half	St Michael	135	38
half	Tesco	135	38
non-dairy	Tesco	280	79
single		212	60
single	BHS	194	228ml 444
	Eden Vale	190	54
	Safeway	200	57
	Sainsbury		1 tbsp 40
	St Ivel	185	52
	St Michael	198	56
	Tesco	188	53
	Waitrose	219	62
soured	Eden Vale	190	54
	Safeway	240	68
	Tesco	188	55
spooning	Eden Vale	363	103
thick double with rum	Tesco	446	126
UHT single	Eden Vale	190	54
whipping	Eden Vale	363	103
whipped	St Michael	379	107
whipping		332	94
whipping	BHS	383	228ml 873
	Eden Vale	363	103

Product	Brand	Calories per 100g/ 100ml	Calories per oz/ pack/ portion
CREAM, whipping	Safeway	410	117
	Sainsbury		1 tbsp unwhipped 65
	St Ivel	380	108
	St Michael	381	108
	Tesco	379	107
Cream cheese	Safeway	500	143
	Sainsbury	458	1 tbsp/½oz 65
	St Ivel	460	130
	Waitrose	818	232
& chives	Waitrose	723	205
& onion	Waitrose	723	205
& pineapple	Waitrose	751	213
Cream crackers		440	125
Cream crackers	BHS	436	124
	Crawford		per biscuit 38
	Jacobs	436	per biscuit 33
	Sainsbury		per biscuit 35
	St Michael	422	per biscuit 37
	Tesco	454	129
	Waitrose	458	130
Cream of asparagus soup	Baxters	62	15oz/425g can 264
Cream of celery soup	Heinz	51	14
condensed (undiluted)	Campbell's	100	28
Cream of chicken soup, canned, ready to serve		58	16
condensed		98	28
condensed, as served		49	14

91

Product	Brand	Calories per 100g/100ml	Calories per oz/pack/portion
Cream of chicken soup	Baxters	57	15oz/425g can 241
	Crosse & Blackwell	63	18
	Heinz	60	17
	Safeway	70	19
	Tesco	54	15
	Waitrose	50	15
condensed (undiluted)	Campbell's	92	26
Cream of Cornish ice cream (242g)	Wall's		per pack 455
sliceable (525g/1 litre)	Wall's		per pack 985
Cream of game soup	Baxters	70	15oz/425g can 296
Cream of leek soup	Baxters	51	15oz/425g can 217
Cream of mushroom soup, canned, ready to serve		*53*	*15*
Cream of mushroom soup, canned (ready to serve)	Baxters	62	15oz/425g can 264
	Crosse & Blackwell	54	15
	Heinz	60	17
	Tesco	55	16
	Waitrose	49	14
condensed (undiluted)	Campbell's	88	25

Product	Brand	Calories per 100g/100ml	Calories per oz/pack/portion
Cream of pheasant soup			15oz/425g can 235
	Baxters	55	
	Frank Cooper	58	15oz can 240
Cream of scampi soup			15oz/425g can 275
	Baxters	65	
	Frank Cooper	63	15oz can 288
Cream of smoked trout soup	Baxters	65	15oz/425g can 277
Cream of tomato soup,			
canned, ready to serve		*55*	*16*
condensed		*123*	*35*
condensed, as served		*62*	*18*
dried		*321*	*91*
dried, as served		*31*	*9*
Cream of tomato soup, canned	Baxters	74	15oz/425g can 319
	Heinz	79	22
	Safeway	70	19
	St Michael	55	16
	Tesco	36	10
	Waitrose	50	15
condensed (undiluted)	Campbell's	131	37
Cream of vegetable soup	Baxters	52	15oz/425g can 221
Cream puffs	St Michael	206	per puff 233
Cream soda sparkling	Cresta	27	7.5
	Corona	26	7.5

Product	Brand	Calories per 100g/ 100ml	Calories per oz/ pack/ portion
Cream style corn	Green Giant	85	24
Cream toffee	Barker Dobson	430	122
Creamed ground rice	Ambrosia	90	26
Creamed macaroni	Ambrosia	96	27
	Safeway	144	45
Creamed macaroni pudding	Waitrose	130	37
Creamed rice	Ambrosia	94	27
	Libby	89	25
	Safeway	144	45
Creamed rice pudding	Waitrose	148	42
Creamed sago	Ambrosia	88	25
Creamed semolina	Ambrosia	90	26
Creamed tapioca	Ambrosia	89	25
	Safeway	144	45
Creamed tapioca pudding	Waitrose	130	37
Creamed tomato soup	Crosse & Blackwell	71	20
Cream-line toffees, bag, box or loose	Callard & Bowser, Nuttall	470	per sweet 40
roll	Callard & Bowser, Nuttall	470	per sweet 23
Creamola custard powder	Rowntree Mackintosh	350	99

Product	Brand	Calories per 100g/ 100ml	Calories per oz/ pack/ portion
Creamola Foam crystals (all flavours)	Rowntree Mackintosh	310	88
Creamola rice	Rowntree Mackintosh	355	101
Creamola steamed or baked pudding mixture	Rowntree Mackintosh	375	106
Creamy chocolate biscuits	Crawford		per biscuit 71
Creamy cucumber dressing	Kraft	494	140
Creamy fudge	Callard & Bowser, Nuttall	420	per bar 230
Creamy instant mash	Yeoman	329	per portion made up with water 61
Creme bears	Cadbury's	435	123
Crème caramel	BHS	83	142g pack 118
	Eden Vale	148	50
	St Ivel	110	31
Creme eggs	Cadbury's	433	123
Crème patisserie doughnuts (4 per pack)	St Michael	347	per doughnut 118
Cresta drinks see Orange, etc			
Crinkle cut crisps	St Michael	545	155
Crisp crackers	Safeway	425	120

Product	Brand	Calories per 100g/ 100ml	Calories per oz/ pack/ portion
Crisp rolls	St Michael	375	per roll 38
Crispbread			
extra thin	Primula	312	per piece 19
light	St Michael	390	per piece 17
new style	Tesco	390	111
rye		*321*	*91*
rye	Sainsbury		per piece 30
rye, extra thin	Sainsbury		per piece 20
wheat	Sainsbury		per piece 30
wheat, starch reduced		*388*	*110*
whole rye	Tesco	375	106
whole wheat with bran	Tesco	360	102
Crispets	Goodies	445	126
Crisps *see also under flavours*			
Crisps:		*533*	*151*
Crisps:	St Michael		
barbecue and onion		533	151
cheese and onion		543	154
crinkle cut		545	155
gammon		530	150
home style		505	143
prawn cocktail		536	152
ready salted		545	155
salt and vinegar		523	148
Crispy vegetable in vinaigrette	St Ivel	70	20
Crofters' thick vegetable soup (as sold)	Knorr	341	97

Product	Brand	Calories per 100g/ 100ml	Calories per oz/ pack/ portion
Croissants	Sainsbury		per croissant 145
Croquette potatoes *see potato croquettes*			
Crumble mix (as sold)	Whitworths	473	5oz pack 671
Crumblebake creams	McVitie		per biscuit 76
Crumpets	Sainsbury		per crumpet 100
Crumpets, Scotch	St Michael	298	84
Crunch creams	Peek Frean	480	per biscuit 57
	Sainsbury		per biscuit 70
Crunch 'n' slim (as sold)	Crookes	460	per meal 230
Crunch nut cake topping	Tesco	495	140
Crunch oat cereal	Safeway	438	125
Crunch sandwich biscuits	St Michael	497	per biscuit 65
Crunchie (large)	Cadbury's	471	134
Crunchy Bran	Allinson	224	64
Crunchy Nut Corn Flakes	Kellogg's	372	105
Crunchy sticks	Safeway	483	138
	Sainsbury	460	25g 115
Crystal fruit flavours	Barker & Dobson	320	91
Cubes (beef)	Beecham	259	73
Cucumber, raw		10	3
Cucumber, pickled dill	Tesco	14	4
Cucumber relish	Tesco	110	31
Cucumber salad	BHS	246	70

Product	Brand	Calories per 100g/ 100ml	Calories per oz/ pack/ portion
Cucumber Sandwich Spread	Heinz	219	62
Cumberland style vegetables with beef	Knorr Hot Pots	361	42g pack 152
Cup Italiano:	Wall's		
choc and nut			each 170
passionfruit cocktail			each 110
raspberry crush			each 120
strawberry			each 125
Cup-a-Soup see under flavours			
Curacao		*311*	*88*
Curd cheese	Sainsbury	141	1 tbsp/½ oz 20
Curls (biscuits)	St Michael	525	per biscuit 38
Curly Wurly	Cadbury's	450	128
Currant bread		*250*	*71*
Currant buns		*302*	*86*
Currant buns	Sainsbury		per bun 135
Currant Crisp biscuits	Peek Frean	440	per biscuit 30
Currants		*243*	*69*
Currants	Safeway	244	69
	Sainsbury	247	1 tbsp/1oz 70
	Tesco	243	69
	Waitrose	243	69
	Whitworths	243	69
Curried beans with sultanas	Heinz	87	25
Curried chicken (canned)	St Michael	120	34

Product	Brand	Calories per 100g/ 100ml	Calories per oz/ pack/ portion
Curried meat		*160*	*45*
Curry, Curry sauce *see also Madras, etc*			
Curry and rice with beef	Snackpot	315	per pot 230
	Vesta	362	per pack 866
Curry and rice with chicken	Snackpot	332	per pot 246
	Vesta	368	per pack 766
Curry concentrate	Lea & Perrins	160	45
Curry Cook-in-Sauce	Homepride	147	376g pack 555
Curry maker, hot mild	Crosse & Blackwell	460 441	130 125
Curry Mix (Colman's) *see Madras, etc*			
Curry Pour Over sauce	Crosse & Blackwell	95	27
Curry powder		*233*	*66*
Curry powder	Tesco	350	99
Curry sauce	Granose	76	22
Curry sauce mix (as sold)	Colman's	350	99
	Knorr	384	109
Curry tomato ketchup	Chef	120	34
Custard (made with egg or powder)		*118*	*33*
Custard, Devon	Ambrosia	103	29
Custard, instant mix (as sold)	Brown & Polson	395	112
Custard, quick	Batchelors	424	per pack 382
Custard creams	BHS	507	144
	Peek Frean	477	per biscuit 61
	Pennywise		per biscuit 60

Product	Brand	Calories per 100g/ 100ml	Calories per oz/ pack/ portion
Custard creams	Sainsbury		per biscuit 55
	St Michael	505	per biscuit 66
	Tesco	459	130
	Waitrose	500	142
Custard mix (made up)	Sainsbury	113	½ pint 320
Custard powder		*354*	*100*
Custard powder	Creamola	350	99
	Fulcreem	330	94
	Tesco	234	66
	Waitrose	352	100
Custard slices (2 per pack)	St Michael	296	per slice 204
Custard tart		*287*	*81*
C-Vit blackcurrant health drink	Beecham Foods	212	60
Cydapple, sparkling	Corona	24	7

Product	Brand	Calories per 100g/ 100ml	Calories per oz/ pack/ portion
Daddies:	HP Foods		
Favourite Sauce		60	17
tomato ketchup		105	30
tomato sauce		66	19
Dads cookies	Chiltonian		per biscuit 43
chocolate chip			per biscuit 43
Dairy Cornish			
ice-cream	Tudor	160	45
Easy Scoop	Tesco	171	48
Dairy cream, whipped	Birds Eye	203	60
Dairy cream and			
chocolate sponge	Birds Eye		1/6 cake 110
Dairy Cream			
desserts	Safeway	250	71
Dairy cream finger			
doughnuts	Sainsbury		each 190
Dairy cream gâteau	Birds Eye		1/6 cake 175
Dairy cream sponge	Birds Eye		1/6 cake 130
Dairy fudge (carton)	Sharps		per pack 1013
			per sweet 42
Dairy Milk chocolate	Cadbury's	526	149
Dairylea cheese			
spread	Kraft	279	79
Damson jam	Hartley's	255	72
Damson preserve,			
Todays Recipe	Robertson's	180	51
Damsons, canned			
(inc. syrup)	Hartley's	95	27
Damsons, raw		*38*	*11*
raw (with stones)		*34*	*9.5*

Product	Brand	Calories per 100g/ 100ml	Calories per oz/ pack/ portion
Damsons			
stewed with sugar		69	20
stewed with sugar and stones		63	18
stewed without sugar		32	9
stewed without sugar (with stones)		29	8
Danbo cheese (45% fat in the dry matter)	Danish	344	98
Dandelion and burdock	Minster	27	7.5
sparkling	Corona	19	5.5
Danish apple dessert	St Michael	312	88
Danish blue cheese	Sainsbury	353	100
	St Ivel	350	99
	St Michael	355	101
(gold)	Tesco	408	116
50% fat in the dry matter	Danish	351	100
60% fat	Danish	379	107
Danish salad	Eden Vale	138	39
Danish shortcake biscuits	Waitrose	529	150
Danish sultana dessert	St Michael	380	108
Danish Toast Slices	Meadow Farm	210	12.5g serving 34
Dansak Classic Curry	Homepride	115	383g pack 440
Dark Satin choc ice	Lyons Maid		each 128

Product	Brand	Calories per 100g/ 100ml	Calories per oz/ pack/ portion
Date and fig dessert bar	Prewetts	261	74
Date and walnut cake	Sainsbury	353	1/6 cake/2oz 200
	Waitrose	310	88
Dates			
dried		*248*	*70*
dried (with stones)		*213*	*60*
Dates			
chopped, sugar rolled	Whitworths	273	77
sugar rolled	Tesco	273	77
Demerara biscuits	Allinson	526	149
Demerara sugar		*394*	*112*
Demerara sugar	Safeway	394	112
	Tesco	394	112
	Waitrose	395	112
	Whitworths	394	112
natural raw cane	Tesco	394	112
Derby cheese	Tesco	388	110
Desiccated coconut		*604*	*171*
Desiccated coconut	Safeway	627	178
	Tesco	604	171
	Whitworths	604	171
Dessert nougat	Callard & Bowser, Nuttall	400	per sweet 56
Dessert topping	Tesco	317	90
Devilled ham paste	Country Pot	190	54
Devon creams	Peek Frean	470	per biscuit 53

Product	Brand	Calories per 100g/100ml	Calories per oz/pack/portion
Devon custard	Ambrosia	103	29
Devon onion soup, thick	Batchelors 5-Minute		per pack 175
Devon toffee bars	Barker & Dobson	430	122
	Palm	416	118
Devon toffees	Parkinsons	416	118
	Sainsbury	458	130
Dextrosol tablets	CPC	343	97
Diabetic			
lemon squash	Rose's	5	1.5
orange squash	Rose's	17	5
Diet Pepsi Cola	Schweppes	0.25	
Digestive biscuits		*471*	*134*
Digestive biscuits	BHS	492	139
	Huntley & Palmers	463	per biscuit 63
	St Michael	499	per biscuit 81
	Tesco	480	136
	Waitrose	504	143
chocolate		*493*	*140*
chocolate	McVitie		per biscuit 130
Goldgrain	Jacobs		per biscuit 59
half-coated	Peek Frean	508	per biscuit 66
milk	Cadbury's	515	146
milk chocolate	Huntley & Palmers	493	per biscuit 62
	Sainsbury		per biscuit 65
	Tesco	518	147
milk chocolate half coat	St Michael	505	per biscuit 65

104

Product	Brand	Calories per 100g/ 100ml	Calories per oz/ pack/ portion
Digestive biscuits			
plain	Cadbury's	465	132
plain chocolate	Huntley & Palmers	490	per biscuit 61
	Sainsbury		per biscuit 70
plain chocolate half coat	St Michael	500	per biscuit 65
small	Sainsbury		per biscuit 45
wheatmeal	McVitie		per biscuit 70
Digestive creams	McVitie		per biscuit 74
	Tesco	510	145
Digestive finger creams	Sainsbury		per biscuit 55
Dijon mustard	Colman's	170	48
Dill & chives Salad Days	Knorr	271	6g pack 16
Dinner balls	Granose	226	64
Dipped Flake	Cadbury's	535	152
Dr. Who bars (all flavours)		381	108
Dogfish fried in batter		265	75
(with waste)		244	69
Dolcelatte	BHS	339	96
	Tesco	340	96
Dolly mixtures	Bassett's	392	111
	Sainsbury	317	90
	St Michael	387	110
Double Decker	Cadbury's	451	128
Double Devon toffees	St Michael	440	125
Double Gloucester cheese	Prewetts	393	111
	Sainsbury	370	105

Product	Brand	Calories per 100g/ 100ml	Calories per oz/ pack/ portion
Double Gloucester *cheese*	St Michael	390	111
	Tesco	367	104
	Waitrose	423	120
Double layer sponge cake	St Michael	272	77
Doughnuts		349	99
Doughnuts (4 per pack)	St Michael	330	each 174
crème patisserie	St Michael	347	each 118
dairy cream	Birds Eye		each 170
finger, dairy cream	Sainsbury		each 190
ring, iced	St Michael	395	112
Dover sole (fresh)	St Michael	95	27
Dracula	Wall's		each 50
Draught cider *see also brand names*			
Draught cider, dry	Taunton	29	1 pint 170
Dried milk *see also brand names and Instant milk, etc*			
Dried milk, skimmed		355	101
whole		490	139
Dried milk, skimmed	Tesco	345	98
skimmed, with vegetable fat	Prewetts	499	141
Dried peas *see Peas*			
Drifter	Rowntree Mackintosh	460	pack (2 biscuits) 230
Drinking chocolate		366	104
Drinking chocolate	BHS	390	111
	Cadbury's	390	111
	Safeway	393	111
	St Michael	366	104

Product	Brand	Calories per 100g/ 100ml	Calories per oz/ pack/ portion
Drinking chocolate	Tesco	390	111
	Waitrose	370	105
	Wander	387	15g/3 heaped tsp 58
(made up)	Sainsbury	70	½ pint (3 tsp + half milk/ water) 200
Dripping, beef		*891*	*253*
Dripping, beef or refined	Tesco	931	264
Dry ginger ale	Britvic	22	6
	Club	26	113ml 30
	Hunts	15	4.5
	Safeway	20–30	6–9
	Schweppes	14	4
	Waitrose	27	8
low calorie	Tesco	6	2
Dry roast peanuts	BHS	544	154
Duck	Waitrose	116	33
Duck, raw			
meat, fat and skin		*430*	*122*
meat only		*122*	*35*
Duck, roast			
meat, fat and skin		*339*	*96*
meat only		*189*	*54*
Duck, roast	Sainsbury	194	1 slice lean/ 1oz 55
Duck with orange soup	Frank Cooper	42	15oz can 192
Duckling, fresh	St Michael	430	122
Dumpling		*211*	*60*

Product	Brand	Calories per 100g/ 100ml	Calories per oz/ pack/ portion
Dumplings in meat sauce	Goblin	120	425g pack 510
Dundee biscuits, milk chocolate	Tesco	483	137
Dundee cake	Sainsbury	388	1/8 cake/2oz 220
	Waitrose	310	88
canned	Lyons	315	per cake 2233
round	St Michael	338	96
Dutch apple slices (2 per pack)	St Michael	212	per slice 190
Dutch finger creams	St Michael	580	per biscuit 48
Dynamo glucose syrup drink	Beechams Foods	140	40

Product	Brand	Calories per 100g/ 100ml	Calories per oz/ pack/ portion
Easy scoop ice cream	Sainsbury	194	1oz/2fl.oz 55
Eccles cakes	Sainsbury		per cake 150
	Waitrose	518	147
all butter	St Michael	390	171
Eclairs		*376*	*107*
Eclairs, chocolate			
(5 per pack)	St Michael	413	each 127
chocolate covered	Waitrose	702	199
dairy cream	Birds Eye		each 130
Edam cheese	Prewetts	304	86
	Sainsbury	300	85
	St Ivel	335	95
	Tesco	303	86
	Waitrose	310	88
Eel			
raw		*168*	*48*
stewed		*201*	*57*
Egg, cheese and bacon flan	Sainsbury	282	¼ flan/3oz 240
Egg custard		*118*	*33*
Egg custard tarts (3 per pack)	St Michael	267	per tart 219
EGGS			
boiled		*147*	*42*
dried		*564*	*160*
fried		*232*	*66*
omelette		*190*	*54*
poached		*155*	*44*
scrambled		*246*	*70*
white, raw		*36*	*10*

109

Product	Brand	Calories per 100g/ 100ml	Calories per oz/ pack/ portion
EGGS			
whole, raw		*147*	*42*
yolk, raw		*339*	*96*
Eggs, fried	Sainsbury		1, size 3 or 4 120
raw, boiled or poached	Sainsbury		1, size 3 or 4 90
Elevenses, milk or plain	Huntley & Palmers	490	per biscuit 92
Emmenthal cheese	Sainsbury	405	115
Endive, raw		*11*	*3*
English herb dressing	Alfonal	370	105
English mustard	Colman's	180	51
Epicure pickles *see Pickled onions, etc*			
Esrom cheese (45% fat in the dry matter)	Danish	344	98
Evaporated milk (whole milk)		*158*	*45*
Evaporated milk	Carnation	165	47
	Ideal	160	45
	Libby	158	45
	Safeway	160	45
	Sainsbury		1 tbsp 45
	Tesco	183	52
	Waitrose	158	45
Exhibition cider,			
dry	Taunton	51	1 pint 300
sweet	Taunton	61	1 pint 360
Extra cereal	Kellogg's	328	93
Extra Strong mints (roll)	Trebor		per pack 145 per sweet 11

Product	Brand	Calories per 100g/ 100ml	Calories per oz/ pack/ portion
Fab	Lyons Maid		each 73
Faggots		*268*	*76*
Faggots, savoury	Sainsbury	282	80
Faggots in rich sauce	Birds Eye	187	13oz pack 690
		182	19oz pack 980
	Brains		each 130
	Ross	180	51
	Sainsbury	200	13oz pack 740
Faggots 'n' Peas	Crosse & Blackwell	112	32
Faggots without sauce	Brains		each 60
Fairy cakes with lemon icing (made up)	Sainsbury		per cake 65
Fairy fruit cake	Sainsbury	341	¼ cake/1½oz 145
Fame	Wall's		each 125
Family Favourites processed cheese (average)	St Ivel	280	79
Fancy gâteau	Sainsbury	450	¹/₅ cake/2oz 255
Fancy iced cakes		*407*	*115*
Fanta lemon or orange	Coca Cola	43	185ml 80, 325ml 140
Farmers thick chicken soup	Batchelors 5-Minute		per pack 233
Farmhouse biscuits	Jacobs	431	per biscuit 34
Farmhouse bran	Weetabix	303	86
Farmhouse crusty bread	St Michael	250	71

Product	Brand	Calories per 100g/ 100ml	Calories per oz/ pack/ portion
Farmhouse pickle	Pan Yan	165	47
Farmhouse pâté	St Michael	300	85
Farmhouse thick vegetable soup	Crosse & Blackwell	53	15
	Heinz	47	13
	Batchelors 5-Minute		per pack 146
Farmhouse yogurt *see yogurt*			
Farola (as sold)	James Marshall	320	91
Ferguzade	Beecham	95	27
Fig bars	Tesco	385	109
Fig biscuits	Prewetts	484	137
Fig rolls	Jacobs	355	per biscuit 51
	Sainsbury		per biscuit 60
Figs, dried, raw		*213*	*60*
stewed with sugar		*136*	*39*
stewed without sugar		*118*	*33*
Figs, green, raw		*41*	*12*
Finger creams, Dutch	St Michael	580	per biscuit 48
Finger wafers, milk	St Michael	482	per wafer 43
plain	St Michael	504	per wafer 45
Fish *see Cod, etc*			
Fish cakes			
fried		*188*	*53*
frozen		*112*	*32*
Fish cakes	BHS	130	per cake 65
	Ross	110	31
	St Michael	100	28

Product	Brand	Calories per 100g/ 100ml	Calories per oz/ pack/ portion
Fish cakes	Tesco	109	31
	Waitrose	215	61
	Sainsbury		per cake, fried 150, grilled 90
cod	Birds Eye		per cake, fried 140
			grilled 90
salmon	Birds Eye		per cake, fried 160
			grilled 100
savoury	Birds Eye		per cake, fried 150
			grilled 95
Fish casserole	St Michael	82	23
Fish fingers			
fried		233	66
frozen		178	50
Fish fingers	BHS		per finger 50
	Ross	180	51
	Safeway	188	53
	Tesco	199	56
	Sainsbury		each, fried 65 grilled 50
cod	Birds Eye		each, fried 65 grilled 55
	St Michael	168	48
Value	Birds Eye		each, fried 55 grilled 45
Fish paste		169	48
Fish pie		128	36
Fish soufflés	St Michael	129	37

Product	Brand	Calories per 100g/ 100ml	Calories per oz/ pack/ portion
Fish steaks in butter sauce	Ross	80	23
Fisherman's pie	BHS	115	33
	Sainsbury	106	30
Five Centre Milk bar	Cadbury's	453	128
Five centre Plain bar	Cadbury's	421	119
5-Minute Soups *see flavours*			
Five Pints milk powder (made up)	St Ivel	46	1 pint 270
Flake	Cadbury's	526	149
Flake, 99	Cadbury's	525	149
Flan case	Lyons	348	per case 480
Flan case, sponge	Tesco	323	92
Flora sunflower dressing	Van den Berghs	493	1 tbsp approx. 75
Florida grapefruit juice (as sold)	Birds Eye	74	1fl.oz 22
(made up)		24	¼ pint 35
orange juice (as sold)	Birds Eye	84	1fl.oz 25
(made up)		30	¼ pint 45
Florida salad	St Ivel	100	28
	Tesco	126	36
	St Michael	205	58
Florida spring vegetable soup (as sold)	Knorr	282	80
FLOUR	Sainsbury	353	1 tbsp/½oz 50
brown	Tesco	333	94
brown (85%)		*327*	*93*
cereal 100%	Allinson	337	96

Product	Brand	Calories per 100g/ 100ml	Calories per oz/ pack/ portion
FLOUR			
farmhouse (plain), 81%	Allinson	351	100
(self-raising), 81%	Allinson	353	100
millstone (plain), 81%	Prewetts	340	96
(self-raising), 81%	Prewetts	353	100
organic 100%	Prewetts	337	96
patent (40%)		*347*	*98*
plain	Safeway	350	100
	Tesco	349	99
	Waitrose	349	99
	Whitworths	350	99
rye (100%)		*335*	*95*
self-raising	Safeway	340	97
	Tesco	349	99
	Waitrose	349	99
	Whitworths	339	96
soya (full fat)		*447*	*127*
(low fat)		*352*	*100*
strong white (unbleached)	Allinson	340	96
	Prewetts	343	97
(unbleached), self-raising	Prewetts	343	97
strong white bread (unbleached)	Prewetts	340	96
superfine plain	Waitrose	349	99
self-raising	Waitrose	349	99
white	Tesco	333	94
white (72%) breadmaking		*337*	*96*

Product	Brand	Calories per 100g/ 100ml	Calories per oz/ pack/ portion
FLOUR			
white household, plain		*350*	*99*
self-raising		*339*	*96*
whole wheat	Tesco	333	94
wholemeal (100%)		*318*	*90*
wholemeal (plain), 100%	Allinson	337	96
	Prewetts	337	96
(self-raising), 100%	Prewetts	339	96
Fondant fancies	Sainsbury		per cake 110
	St Michael	339	per cake 112
Force wheat flakes	A.C. Fincken	360	102
Forerib *see Beef*			
Forestier pâté	BHS	340	96
Fox's Glacier Fruits	Rowntree Mackintosh	365	per sweet 11
Fox's Glacier Mints	Rowntree Mackintosh	380	per sweet 12
Frankfurter, family	St Michael	274	78
Frankfurters		*274*	*78*
Frankfurters	Sainsbury		1 sm/1oz 70 1/3oz 210
Freeze Pops	Tesco	38	11
French beans canned	Waitrose	18	5
whole	Birds Eye	35	10
French bread pizza	BHS	238	per pizza 310
	Birds Eye		per pizza 330

116

product	Brand	Calories per 100g/ 100ml	Calories per oz/ pack/ portion
french bread pizza de luxe	Ross	210	60
	Birds Eye		per pizza 360
french dressing		658	187
french dressing classic	Heinz	519	147
	Kraft	423	120
oil free	Waistline	13	4
french jam sandwich	BHS	448	262g cake 1173
	Sainsbury	329	1/7 cake/ 1½oz 140
	Waitrose	360	102
french onion soup canned	Baxters	14	15oz/425g can 59
	Crosse & Blackwell	18	5
	Frank Cooper	17	15oz can 80
dried (as sold)	Batchelors 5-Minute		per pack 99
	Knorr	328	93
dried (made up)	Maggi Quick Cook	18	5
with cheese and croûtons	Cup-a-Soup Special	305	per portion 58
french style onion soup (as sold)	Tesco	234	66
fresca	Coca Cola		325ml negl.
fresh cream dessert	Eden Vale	143	41
fresh cream dessert, chocolate	St Ivel	154	44
fruit	St Ivel	148	42

Product	Brand	Calories per 100g/ 100ml	Calories per oz/ pack/ portion
Fresh cream trifle	Sainsbury		sm tub 230
	Tesco	176	50
Fricassée	Granose	120	34
Fried bread		*558*	*158*
Fried chicken spread	Princes	219	62
Fried rice, special	Birds Eye		per pack 450
Frikaletts	Granose	119	34
Frosted creams	Pennywise		per biscuit 59
Frosties	Kellogg's	351	100
Fruit and bran bar	Prewetts	204	58
Fruit and Nut, Bourneville	Cadbury's	464	132
milk	Cadbury's	467	132
Fruit and nut biscuits	Allinson	514	146
Fruit and nut dessert bar	Prewetts	307	87
Fruit and nut toffees	Parkinsons	416	118
Fruit and nuts, exotic	Tesco	283	80
Fruit Bonbons	Pascall	368	104
Fruit bon-bons	Sainsbury	335	95
Fruit buns, spiced	St Michael	285	81
Fruit cake			
plain		*354*	*100*
rich		*332*	*94*
rich, iced		*352*	*100*
Fruit cake			
country style	Waitrose	367	104
home style	Sainsbury	370	1/7 cake/2oz 210

Product	Brand	Calories per 100g/ 100ml	Calories per oz/ pack/ portion
Fruit cake			
iced	Sainsbury	326	¹/₆ small/¹/₅ large/2oz 185
rich, all butter	St Michael	353	100
rich, iced top	St Michael	310	88
Fruit chews (bag)	St Michael	381	108
(stick pack)	St Michael	368	104
Fruit chocolate bon-bons	Parkinsons	404	115
Fruit cocktail	BHS	76	22
	Libby	79	22
	Waitrose	95	27
(drained)	Tesco	74	21
(including syrup)	Sainsbury	75	1 tbsp/1oz 21
in fruit juice	John West	47	13
in syrup	John West	60	17
Fruit cocktail jelly (as sold)	Chivers	280	79
Fruit cocktail sundae	Eden Vale	126	36
Fruit cocktail trifle	BHS	126	113g pack 142
Fruit desserts	Sainsbury		sm. tub 150
Fruit desserts, fresh cream	St Ivel	148	42
Fruit digestives	Huntley & Palmers	450	per biscuit 50
Fruit drops, assorted	St Michael	360	102
Fruit drops, old-fashioned	Parkinsons	378	107

Product	Brand	Calories per 100g/ 100ml	Calories per oz/ pack/ portion
Fruit finger buns, iced	St Michael	309	88
Fruit flan fillings *see under flavours*			
Fruit flavoured assortment (sweets)	St Michael	350	99
Fruit flavoured candy products	Goodies	532	151
Fruit flavoured drops	Bensons	320	91
Fruit fool	Eden Vale	238	67
Fruit gums		*172*	*49*
Fruit Gums	Rowntree Mackintosh	170	per tube 65
Fruit jellies (sweets)	BHS	300	85
	Sainsbury	335	95
	Selesta	306	87
	Waitrose	258	73
Fruit lumps	Parkinsons	381	108
Fruit malt loaf	St Michael	266	75
Fruit mousse, Wizard	St Ivel	180	51
Fruit passionata Italiano	Wall's		558g/1 litre pack 880
Fruit pastilles	Barker & Dobson	253	72
	Pascall	312	88
	Rowntree Mackintosh	320	per tube 130
	St Michael	344	98
Fruit pie, individual, with pastry *top and bottom*		*369*	*105*
with pastry top		*180*	*51*

Product	Brand	Calories per 100g/100ml	Calories per oz/pack/portion
Fruit pie filling, canned		*95*	*27*
Fruit pie filling, canned brands *see under flavours*			
Fruit pudding, rich	Sainsbury	336	10½oz can 1000
Fruit salad	BHS	207	59
canned		95	27
canned	Waitrose	95	27
canned drained	Tesco	94	27
Fruit salad sweets	Trebor		per sweet 14
Fruit sauce	Lea & Perrins	120	34
	Tesco	67	19
Fruit shortcake biscuits	BHS	476	135
	McVitie		per biscuit 50
	Sainsbury		per biscuit 35
	Tesco	461	131
	Waitrose	472	134
Fruit soufflés	St Ivel	160	45
Fruit sweets, assorted	St Michael	378	107
Fruit thins	Parkinsons	378	107
Fruit trifle, individual	St Michael	158	45
large	St Michael	165	47
Fruity crisp	Sainsbury	423	¹/s cake/1oz 120
Fruity ketchup	Pan Yan	165	47
Fruity sauce	HP Foods	90	26
	O.K. (Colman's)	90	26

121

Product	Brand	Calories per 100g/ 100ml	Calories per oz/ pack/ portion
Fruity sauce	Safeway	100	28
Fry's Chocolate Cream	Cadbury's	414	117
Fry's Turkish Delight	Cadbury's	361	102
Fudge	Cadbury's	440	125
	Tesco	385	88
Fulfilling sandwich fillings:	Armour		
chopped chicken with peppers		147	42
chopped ham and egg		120	34
cured beef and onion		135	38
smoked mackerel		228	65
spreadable corned beef		146	41
Funny Faces	Wall's		each 75
Funny Feet	Wall's		each 85
Fussell's Blue Butterfly condensed milk	Nestlé	267	76
Fussell's Golden Butterfly sterilized cream	Nestlé	233	66
Fynbo cheese (45% fat in the dry matter)	Danish	344	98

Product	Brand	Calories per 100g/ 100ml	Calories per oz/ pack/ portion
Galaxy	Mars	538	50g 269, 70g 376, 100g 539, 150g 806
Game consommé	Baxters	12	15oz/425g can 49

Game soup *see also Cream of game*

Product	Brand	Calories per 100g/ 100ml	Calories per oz/ pack/ portion
Game soup	Frank Cooper	42	15oz can 180
Gammon	Waitrose	324	92
boiled	Sainsbury	176	1oz lean 50
Danish D shaped joint	St Michael	206	58
joint, boiled			
lean and fat		*269*	*76*
lean only		*167*	*47*
joint, raw (lean and fat)		*236*	*67*
rashers, grilled			
lean and fat		*228*	*65*
lean only		*172*	*49*
rind-on joint, smoked	St Michael	246	70
smoked sliced	St Michael	269	76
Gammon steaks (uncooked)	Danepak	250	71
Canadian-style	St Michael	182	52
Danish D shaped	St Michael	206	58
Danish round unsmoked	St Michael	173	49
Gammon and pork steaklets (as sold)	Tiffany's	240	4oz steaklet 265

Product	Brand	Calories per 100g/ 100ml	Calories per oz/ pack/ portion
Gammon crisps	St Michael	530	150
Garden mint sauce	Pan Yan	45	13
Garden peas *see Peas*			
Garden vegetable soup, thick (made up)	Chef Box	25	7
Garibaldi biscuits	Peek Frean	364	per biscuit 30
	Pennywise		per biscuit 33
	Sainsbury		per biscuit 30
	Tesco	380	108
	Waitrose	380	108
half coat	Peek Frean	392	per biscuit 83
Garlic salt	Tesco	30	8.5
Garlic sausage	BHS	302	86
Gelatin		*338*	*96*
Gelatine	Davis	105	30
Genoa cake	Sainsbury	400	$^1/_7$ cake/ 1½oz 170
Genoese fancies	BHS	367	per fancy 103
German mustard	Colman's	135	38
Gherkins, cocktail	Tesco	11	3
Gherkins, pickled	Crosse & Blackwell	2	
	Epicure	17	5
	Haywards	5	1.5
Ginger, ground		*258*	*73*
Ginger, ground	Tesco	350	99
	Whitworths	258	73
Ginger ale, American	Britvic	34	9.5
	Club	35	113ml 40, 185ml 65

Product	Brand	Calories per 100g/100ml	Calories per oz/pack/portion
Ginger ale, American	Hunts	39	11
	Idris	28	8
	Safeway	20–30	6–9
	Schweppes	21	6
	Tesco	28	8
	Waitrose	28	8
low calorie	Club	negl.	negl.
	Hunts	1	
	Slimsta	4	1
	Tesco	6	2
slimline	Schweppes	0.35	
Ginger ale, American dry	Sainsbury	14	125ml/¼ pint 20
low calorie	Sainsbury	1.5	125ml/¼ pint 2
Ginger ale, dry	Britvic	22	6
	Club	26	113ml 30
	Hunts	15	4.5
	Safeway	20–30	6–9
	Schweppes	14	4
	Tesco	18	5
	Waitrose	27	8
low calorie	Tesco	6	2
Ginger beer	Britvic	41	12
	Club	29	185ml 55
	Corona	29	8
	Schweppes	31	9
	Waitrose	44	13
(canned)	Safeway	49	14
Old English	Idris	47	13
Ginger biscuits	Allinson	395	112

Product	Brand	Calories per 100g/ 100ml	Calories per oz/ pack/ portion
Ginger cake, Scotch	Sainsbury	300	1/7 cake/2oz 170
Ginger cordial	Schweppes	91	26
Ginger creams	BHS	493	140
	Safeway	492	140
	Sainsbury		per biscuit 70
Ginger crunch	Pennywise		per biscuit 26
Ginger nuts		*456*	*129*
Ginger nuts	McVitie		per biscuit 44
	Tesco	431	122
Ginger pear bar	Granose	315	89
Ginger punch (undiluted)	Corona	109	31
Ginger snaps	Crawford		per biscuit 33
	Peek Frean	434	per biscuit 29
	Sainsbury		per biscuit 35
	St Michael	429	per biscuit 33
Ginger thins	BHS	465	132
	Sainsbury		per biscuit 25
Gingerbread		*373*	*106*
Gingerbread	St Michael	308	87
Gingerbread men	Sainsbury		per man 145
	Waitrose	444	126
Gingerella biscuits	Chiltonian	425	per biscuit 28
Gipsy creams	McVitie		per biscuit 82
Glacé cherries		*212*	*60*
Glacé cherries	Safeway	318	90
	Tesco	282	80
	Waitrose	212	60
	Whitworths	212	60

Product	Brand	Calories per 100g/ 100ml	Calories per oz/ pack/ portion
Glacé mints	Barker & Dobson	320	91
Glacier Fruits, Fox's	Rowntree Mackintosh	365	per sweet 11
Glacier Mints, Fox's	Rowntree Mackintosh	380	per sweet 12
Glees, chocolate	Mars		per pack 190
Glees, jam	Mars		per pack 170
Glengarry biscuits	Crawford		per biscuit 50
Glucodin	Farley	340	96
Glucose liquid, BP		*318*	*90*
Gluten-free biscuits	Farley	535	per biscuit 54
Gold margarine	St Ivel	375	106
Gold Seal ice cream:	Lyons Maid		
black cherry		119	35
caramel toffee		114	34
choc almond		140	41
choc nut sundae			each 94
coffee hazelnut		106	31
mint choc chip		105	31
mint choc sundae			each 91
raspberry peach sundae		106	31
raspberry sundae			each 77
vanilla choc flake		120	35
Gold Spinner processed cheese	St Ivel	280	79
Golden Crumble	McVitie		per biscuit 40
Golden crunch creams	BHS	511	145
	Safeway	511	145

Product	Brand	Calories per 100g/ 100ml	Calories per oz/ pack/ portion
Golden Cup	Rowntree Mackintosh	475	small pack 105
Golden Grains	Prewetts	376	107
Golden Grill	Fletchers	105	30
Golden lentil soup	Batchelors 5-Minute		per pack 207
Golden mints	BHS	376	150g pack 564
Golden orange	Lyons Maid		each 57
Golden pea with ham soup (undiluted)	Granny's	57	16
Golden Shred	Robertson's	251	7
Golden syrup *see Syrup*			
Golden syrup butter sponge pudding (as sold)	Tiffany's	305	$\frac{1}{4}$ pudding 275
Golden Toffee	Rowntree Mackintosh	460	per sweet 30
Golden vanilla ice cream			
bar	Wall's		each 85
block	Wall's	175	157g pack 275 241g pack 420
sliceable	Wall's	175	litre pack 915
soft scoop	Wall's	922	2-litre pack 1845
tub	Wall's		each 105
Golden vegetable soup, canned condensed	St Michael	37	10
(undiluted)	Campbell's	41	12

Product	Brand	Calories per 100g/100ml	Calories per oz/pack/portion
Golden vegetable soup			
dried (as sold)	Batchelors		
	Cup-a-Soup	360	per portion 72
	Batchelors		
	5-Minute		per pack 217
	Knorr		
	Quick	424	120
dried (made up)	Chef Box	29	8
low calorie	Slim-a-Soup		per portion 37
	Waistline	17	5
Golden Wheat biscuits	Jacobs	450	per biscuit 42
Goldgrain digestive biscuits	Jacobs	490	per biscuit 59
Good Start	Libby	35	10
Goose, roast		*319*	*90*
Gooseberries	Safeway	90	26
canned (inc. syrup)	Hartley's	80	23
	Sainsbury	75	1tbsp/1oz 21
fresh or frozen	Sainsbury	4	1tbsp/1oz 1
Goosberries, green			
raw		*17*	*5*
stewed with sugar		*50*	*14*
stewed without sugar		*14*	*4*
Gooseberries, ripe, raw		*37*	*10*
Gooseberry crumble, baked	Tiffany's	230	¼ crumble 260
Gooseberry flan filling	Armour	89	25
Gooseberry pie filling	Tesco	95	27

Product	Brand	Calories per 100g/ 100ml	Calories per oz/ pack/ portion
Gooseberry slice	St Michael	254	72
Gooseberry tarts	Sainsbury		per tart 275
Gorgonzola cheese	Sainsbury	335	95
Gouda cheese	Sainsbury	353	100
	St Ivel	370	105
	Tesco	342	97
	Waitrose	338	96
Goulash	Granose	54	15
Goulash Casserole Mix (as sold)	Colman's	275	78
Granary bread	St Michael	237	67
Grand Marnier bars	St Michael	467	132
Granola	Macfarlane Lang		per biscuit 57
Grape juice drink			
red	H.P. Bulmer	46	13
sparkling	Shloer	49	14
sparkling red	Shloer	49	14
white	H.P. Bulmer	46	13
Grapefruit, canned		*60*	*17*
Grapefruit, canned			
segments, drained	Tesco	63	18
segments (inc. syrup)	Sainsbury	40	1tbsp/1oz 11
segments in juice	Libby	30	8.5
segments in natural juice, drained	Tesco	34	9.5
segments in natural juice	John West	42	12
segments in syrup	John West	59	17

Product	Brand	Calories per 100g/ 100ml	Calories per oz/ pack/ portion
Grapefruit, canned segments with sugar (inc. syrup)	Sainsbury	75	1tbsp/1oz 21
Grapefruit, fresh, raw		*22*	*6*
raw (whole fruit)		*11*	*3*
Grapefruit, fresh	Sainsbury	11	½ med./5oz 15
Grapefruit and pineapple drink (undiluted)	Idris	105	30
	Quosh	105	30
Grapefruit barley water	Robinsons	105	30
Grapefruit 'C' reduced calories	Libby	30	8.5
sweetened	Libby	58	16
Grapefruit crush	Slimsta	5	1.5
Grapefruit drink low calorie	Chekwate	13	4
sparkling (bottled)	Tango	45	13
sparkling (canned)	Hunts	40	11
	Tango	42	12
whole (undiluted)	Corona	101	29
	Idris	101	29
Grapefruit drink with pineapple juice (undiluted)	Corona	105	30
Grapefruit juice, canned, sweetened		*38*	*11*
unsweetened		*31*	*9*

131

Product	Brand	Calories per 100g/ 100ml	Calories per oz/ pack/ portion
Grapefruit juice	Britvic	52	15
	Club	62	113ml 70
	Heinz	66	19
	Prewetts	40	11
	Safeway	14	4
	Schweppes	60	17
	Waitrose	20	6
fresh	BHS	36	10
natural	Tesco	42	12
sweetened	Hunts	62	18
	Libby	38	11
	Sainsbury	53	¼ pint 75
	Tesco	49	14
Texas pink	St Michael	30	8.5
UHT	BHS	40	11
unsweetened	Libby	31	9
	Sainsbury	39	¼ pint 55
Grapefruit marmalade	Baxters	247	12oz/340g jar 840
Grapefruit museli yogurt	Country Prize	83	24
Grapefruit Rise and Shine	Kellogg's	327 (dry)	4fl.oz/114ml 49
Grapefruit squash	Sainsbury	18	½ pint diluted from 4 tbsp 50
Grapefruit whole fruit drink	Robinsons	95	27
Grapenuts		*355*	*101*
Grapes	Sainsbury	53	15

Product	Brand	Calories per 100g/ 100ml	Calories per oz/ pack/ portion
Grapes, black			
raw		61	17
raw (whole grapes)		51	14
Grapes, white			
raw		63	18
raw (whole grapes)		60	17
Gravy and lean roast beef	Birds Eye	84	4oz pack 95
Gravy and roast chicken	Birds Eye	84	8oz pack 190
Gravy and roast leg of pork	Birds Eye	123	8oz pack 280
Gravy browning	Fletchers	99	28
Gravy cubes	Knorr	353	9g cube 32
Gravy mix	Tesco	259	73
Gravy pot, concentrated	Colman's	535	152
Gravy with sliced roast beef	Ross	100	28
Green beans			
canned cut (drained)	Tesco	14	4
canned sliced	Safeway	3	negl.
dried	Whitworths	143	41
fresh, frozen or canned and drained	Sainsbury	18	1 tbsp/1oz 5
frozen	Ross	35	10
	Waitrose	14	4
frozen sliced	Birds Eye	28	8
	Tesco	14	4

Product	Brand	Calories per 100g/ 100ml	Calories per oz/ pack/ portion
Green pea soup, thick (dried, made up)	Sainsbury	28	½ pint 80
Greengages			
raw		47	13
raw (with stones)		45	13
stewed with sugar		75	21
stewed with sugar (with stones)		72	20
stewed without sugar		40	11
stewed without sugar (with stones)		38	11
Grillsteaks	Ross	320	91
Ground almonds, rice, etc, see *Almonds, Rice, etc*			
Ground rice pudding, creamed	Ambrosia	90	26
Groundnut oil	Safeway	900	255
	Waitrose	885	262
Grouse, roast		173	49
(with bone)		114	32
Gruyère cheese	Sainsbury	423	120
	Tesco	434	123
Gruyère spread	Tesco	395	112
Guavas, canned		60	17

Product	Brand	Calories per 100g/ 100ml	Calories per oz/ pack/ portion
Hacks medicated products	Barker & Dobson	320	91
HADDOCK			
breaded (frozen)	BHS	149	42
chunky	BHS	76	per pack 187
cutlets (frozen)	Waitrose	70	20
Faroese fillets (fresh)	St Michael	75	21
fillet (frozen)	Birds Eye	71	20
fillets (frozen)	BHS	80	23
	Ross	80	23
	Waitrose	95	27
in breadcrumbs (as sold)	Ross	120	34
poached in milk	Sainsbury	106	30
fried		*174*	*49*
(with bones)		*160*	*45*
fried (frozen)	Waitrose	176	50
frozen	BHS Safeway	80	23
golden (fresh or frozen)	Sainsbury	70	20
golden cutlets	St Michael	83	24
raw		*73*	*21*
skinless boneless fillets (fresh)	St Michael	75	21
smoked	Sainsbury	106	30
buttered	Birds Eye	106	30
frozen	BHS	80	23

Product	Brand	Calories per 100g/ 100ml	Calories per oz/ pack/ portion
HADDOCK			
smoked fillets	Ross	80	23
	St Michael	83	24
(frozen)	Waitrose	98	28
with butter	Ross	90	26
	St Michael	83	24
smoked steamed		*101*	*29*
smoked steamed			
(with bones and skin)		*66*	*19*
steaks	Birds Eye		per steak 80
crispy	Birds Eye		per steak 175 deep fried 200, shallow fried 180
in butter sauce	Ross	80	23
in crisp crunch			
crumb	Birds Eye		per steak 185 fried 210 grilled or baked 185
steamed		*98*	*28*
steamed (with bones and skin)		*75*	*21*
Haddock and prawn crumble	BHS	150	43
Haddock in breadcrumbs, bakeable	St Michael	170	48
chunky or small fillets or 2lb bag	St Michael	119	34
grilled or fried (with a little oil)	Sainsbury	212	60

136

Product	Brand	Calories per 100g/ 100ml	Calories per oz/ pack/ portion
Haddock in parsley sauce	Birds Eye		per pack 175
Haggis, boiled		*310*	*88*
Haggis, Scottish	Baxters	170	14½oz/411g can 699
Halibut			
raw		*92*	*26*
steamed		*131*	*37*
steamed (with bones and skin)		*99*	*28*
Halibut steaks	Waitrose	130	37
Ham	Waitrose	434	123
canned		*120*	*34*
canned	Sainsbury	123	1 thin slice/ 1oz 35
canned Danish	St Michael	120	34
mild cure	BHS	141	40
Old English	BHS	190	54
sliced	Sainsbury	159	1 slice/1oz 45
sliced and thin			
sliced Danish	St Michael	130	37
sliced honey roast	St Michael	173	49
sliced roasted	St Michael	220	62
sliced smoked mildcure	St Michael	160	45
sliced smoked spiced	St Michael	220	62
Ham, leek and cheese pie (1½lb), baked	Tiffany's	235	¼ pie 420
Ham, turkey and vegetable soup (undiluted)	Campbell's Main-Course	55	16

137

Product	Brand	Calories per 100g/ 100ml	Calories per oz/ pack/ portion
Ham and beef paste	Shippams	200	57
Ham and beef roll	Crosse & Blackwell	226	64
Ham and cheese Toast Topper	Heinz	195	55
Ham and chicken roll	Crosse & Blackwell	220	62
Ham and mushroom deep dish pizza	St Michael	207	59
Ham and mushroom pie	Safeway	295	85
Ham and mushroom pizza	Birds Eye	242	265g pizza 640
(5, 7 or 9in)	Ross	220	62
Ham and pineapple pizza (5in)	Ross	220	62
Ham and tongue roll	Crosse & Blackwell	270	77
Ham sausage	BHS	161	46
Bavarian	St Michael	160	45
Ham spread	Princes	229	65
	St Michael	300	85
	Shippams	195	55
Ham stock cubes	Knorr	247	9.5 cube 23
Ham/cured pork shoulder	Armour	111	31
Hamburgers *see also Beefburgers, Burgers*			
Hamburgers	Danish Prime	210	60
(canned)	Waitrose	162	46

Product	Brand	Calories per 100g/ 100ml	Calories per oz/ pack/ portion
Hamburgers			
American	Ross	320	91
in gravy (canned)	Tesco	145	41
with onion	Kraft		each, well grilled 80
	Ross	260	74
with onions and			
gravy	Goblin	140	425g pack 595
Hare, stewed		*192*	*54*
(with bone)		*139*	*39*
Haricot beans (raw)	Safeway	258	73
Harvest Crunch	Quaker Oats	428	121
Harvest vegetable and chicken soup	Batchelors 5-Minute		per pack 217
Hash browns (as sold)	Ross	80	23
Havarti cheese	St Michael	421	119
	Tesco	420	119
45% fat in dry matter	Danish	318	90
60% fat in dry matter	Danish	414	117
Hazel nuts		*380*	*107*
(with shells)		*137*	*39*
Hazel nuts	Whitworths	639	181
Hazelnut biscuits	Allinson	506	143
Hazelnut kernels	Sainsbury	388	110
Hazelnut roll	Tesco	427	121
Hazelnut toffee nougat	St Michael	490	139

Product	Brand	Calories per 100g/ 100ml	Calories per oz/ pack/ portion
Hazelnut yogurt/ yoghurt		106	30
Hazelnut yogurt/ yoghurt	Prize	87	25
	Sainsbury	106	sm. tub/ ¼ pint 150
	Ski	100	28
	Waitrose	95	27
Hazelnuts, roasted	Tesco	750	213
Heart			
lamb, raw		119	34
ox, raw		108	31
ox, stewed		179	51
pig, raw		93	26
sheep, roast		237	67
Hereford style vegetables with beef	Knorr Hot Pots	357	45g pack 161
Herring			
fried		234	66
fried (with bones)		206	58
grilled		199	56
grilled (with bones)		135	38
raw		234	66
Herring	Sainsbury	229	65
baked (frozen)	Waitrose	190	54
boned (frozen)	Waitrose	236	67
fillets in savoury sauce	John West	118	33
fillets in tomato sauce	John West	138	39
in tomato sauce, Scotch	Crosse & Blackwell	154	44

140

Product	Brand	Calories per 100g/ 100ml	Calories per oz/ pack/ portion
Herring roe, soft			
fried		*244*	*69*
raw		*80*	*23*
Highland lentil soup			87g/1½ pint
(as sold)	Knorr	339	pack 295
Highlander's Broth	Baxters	35	15oz/425g can 147
Hi-Juice	Schweppes	50	14
Home style crisps	St Michael	505	143
Home style fruit cake	Sainsbury	370	¹/₇ cake/2oz 210
Honey			
comb		*281*	*80*
in jars		*288*	*82*
Honey	BHS	304	86
	Gales	310	88
	Safeway	284	81
	Sainsbury	317	1 tbsp/1oz 90
	St Michael	290	82
	Tesco	289	82
Honey Bear spread	Bear Brand	290	82
Honey biscuits	Allinson	456	129
Honeycomb Crunch	St Michael	614	174
Horlicks		*396*	*112*
Horlicks	Beecham	393	111
tablets	Beecham	387	each 6.5
Horseradish, creamed	Colman's	210	60
Horseradish, raw		*59*	*17*
Horseradish cream	Tesco	187	53
Horseradish mustard	Colman's	140	40

Product	Brand	Calories per 100g/ 100ml	Calories per oz/ pack/ portion
Horseradish relish	Colman's	100	28
Horseradish sauce	Safeway	82	23
	Sainsbury	88	1 tbsp/1oz 25
	Tesco	125	35
creamed	Colman's	210	59
	Sainsbury	194	1 tbsp/1oz 55
Hot chocolate mix (as sold)	Carnation	379	28g sachet 108
Hot dog sausages (canned)	Tesco	182	52
Hot Oat Cereal	Safeway	400	114
Hot pot		*114*	*32*
Hot Pots (Knorr) *see Cornish, etc*			
Hotel biscuits	Sainsbury		per biscuit 9.5
Hovis bread		*228*	*65*
Hovis bread	St Michael	230	65
HP Sauce	HP Foods	75	21
Humbugs, old fashioned	Parkinsons	386	109
Hundreds and thousands	Tesco	375	106
Hycal (blackcurrant, lemon, orange, raspberry)	Beecham Foods	244	69

Product	Brand	Calories per 100g/ 100ml	Calories per oz/ pack/ portion
Ice cream, dairy		*167*	*47*
non-dairy		*165*	*47*
Ice cream, branded packs *see under flavours or names, eg Easy scoop; Vanilla*			
Ice cream roll, value	Birds Eye		1/6 roll 55
Iced all butter madeira sandwich cake	St Michael	389	110
Iced cakes, fancy		*407*	*115*
Iced fruit cake	Sainsbury	326	1/6 small/ 1/15 large/ 2oz 185
Iced fruit finger buns	St Michael	309	88
Iced Gems	Peek Frean	408	per biscuit 5
Iced ring biscuits	Waitrose	448	127
Iced ring doughnuts	St Michael	395	112
Iced sponge (marzipan) roll	Tesco	416	118
Iced top all butter madeira Xmas cake	St Michael	413	117
Iced top rich fruit cake	St Michael	310	88
Icing sugar, sifter	Whitworths	388	110
Ideal evaporated milk	Nestlé	160	45
Ideal sauce	Heinz	115	33
Indian tonic water	Britvic	31	9
	Club	26	113ml 30, 185ml 50
	Hunts	23	6.5
	Idris	24	7
	Tesco	25	7

143

Product	Brand	Calories per 100g/ 100ml	Calories per oz/ pack/ portion
Indian Tonic Water			
low calorie	Club	negl.	negl.
	Hunts	4	1
	Slimsta	4	1
	Tesco	6	2
Instant dessert,			
chocolate (made up)	Safeway	137	39
all other flavours	Safeway	138	39
Instant mashed			
potatoes	Safeway	332	94
Instant milk	Safeway	352	100
	Waitrose	328	93
(made up)	Wander	335	1 pint 190
Instant mix custard	Brown & Polson	395	112
Instant potato powder		*318*	*90*
(made up)		*70*	*20*
Irish stew		*124*	*35*
(with bones)		*114*	*32*
Irish stew (canned)	Goblin	100	425g can 425
	Sainsbury	88	15oz can 375
	Tesco	124	35
Irn Bru	Barr	40	11
Italian salad	Eden Vale	131	37
Italian Garlic dressing	Kraft	571	162
Italian style sausage pizza	St Michael	214	61
Italian tomato and vegetable soup	Batchelors 5-Minute		per pack 148
Italiano (Wall's) *see under flavours*			

144

Product	Brand	Calories per 100g/ 100ml	Calories per oz/ pack/ portion
Jaffa assortment (sweets)	St Michael	350	99
Jaffa biscuits, milk chocolate	Tesco	420	119
Jaffa cakes	BHS	390	per biscuit 47
	McVitie		per biscuit 50
	Sainsbury		per biscuit 50
Jaffa orange dessert	St Michael	114	32
Jaffa orange juice	St Michael	33	9.5
Jaffa orange yoghurt	St Michael	85	24
Jam *see also under Strawberry, etc*			
Jam			
fruit with edible seeds		*261*	*74*
stone fruit		*261*	*74*
Jam	Sainsbury	265	1 tbsp/1oz 75
Jam and cream sandwich biscuits	Tesco	476	135
Jam and vanilla roll:	Sainsbury		
large		300	1/8 roll/1oz 85
small		353	1/6 roll/1oz 100
Jam and vanilla sponge sandwich	Lyons	361	per cake 892
Jam and vanilla Swiss roll	Lyons	333	per roll 627
Jam pudding (foil basin)	Sainsbury		whole 715
Jam Rings	Pennywise		per biscuit 63
Jam roll boxed	St Michael	374	106

Product	Brand	Calories per 100g/ 100ml	Calories per oz/ pack/ portion
Jam roll			
junior	Sainsbury		per roll 70
large	Sainsbury	282	¹/₈ roll/1oz 80
small	Sainsbury	300	¹/₆ roll/1oz 85
Jam roly poly	Tiffany's	315	¼ roll 265
Jam sandwich biscuits	Tesco	469	133
Jam sandwich creams	Safeway	475	136
	St Michael	475	per biscuit 71
Jam Swiss roll	BHS	259	177g roll 458
	Lyons	298	per roll 557
	St Michael	290	82
	Waitrose	324	92
Jam tarts		384	109
Jam tarts	BHS	403	per tart 141
	Lyons	412	per tart 99
	Sainsbury		per tart 130
	Waitrose	480	136
mini	Tesco	466	132
Jam vanilla Swiss roll	Waitrose	367	104
Jamaica ginger cake	Lyons	328	per cake 1030
	Waitrose	321	91
Jamaica rum and raisin Soft Scoop	Wall's		2 litre pack 2045
Jamboree mallows	Peek Frean	382	per biscuit 77
Jarlsberg cheese	Sainsbury	335	95
	Tesco	353	100
Jellies (dessert/table) *see also under flavours*			
Jellies (dessert/table) made with milk		86	24

146

Product	Brand	Calories per 100g/ 100ml	Calories per oz/ pack/ portion
Jellies (dessert/table)			
made with water		59	17
packet, cubes (as sold)		259	73
Jellies (dessert/table)	Rowntree		
as sold	Mackintosh	290	82
	Safeway	259	73
made up	Sainsbury		pkt 300
	Tesco	59	17
Jellies (preserves) see under Redcurrant, etc			
Jelly babies	Bassett's	342	97
	Sainsbury	335	95
Jelly beans	Sainsbury	335	95
Jelly bears	Sainsbury	317	90
Jelly Creams see under flavours			
Jelly diamonds	Tesco	360	102
Jellytots	Rowntree		
	Mackintosh	345	sm. bag 170
Jersey Creams	Peek Frean	475	per biscuit 57
Jersey potatoes (canned)	Waitrose	74	21
Jersey Royal new potatoes	BHS	53	15
Juice bar:			
grapefruit	Lyons Maid		each 45
orange/pineapple			each 47
Juicy Jellies	Callard &		
	Bowser	310	per sweet 32
Jumboburgers	Ross	240	68
Junior choc roll:			
caramel	Lyons	426	per roll 107
raspberry		361	per roll 97

Product	Brand	Calories per 100g/ 100ml	Calories per oz/ pack/ portion
Junior rolls,			
chocolate	Sainsbury		per roll 120
chocolate with choc.			
buttercream	St Michael	465	per roll 133
covered buttercream	St Michael	446	per roll 156
jam	Sainsbury		per roll 70
Junior Swiss rolls	BHS	415	per roll 145
Jusoda orange drink	Barr	35	10
Just Bake chips	St Michael	208	59

Product	Brand	Calories per 100g/100ml	Calories per oz/pack/portion
K9	Wall's		each 50
Kashmir beef curry			
Knoodles	Knorr	368	104
Kashmir chicken soup	Frank Cooper	42	15oz can 180
Kedgeree		*151*	*43*
Kedgeree	St Michael	150	43
Kennet biscuits	Huntley & Palmers	466	per biscuit 46
Kia-Ora drinks *see Lemon, etc*			
Kidney			
lamb, fried		*155*	*44*
lamb, raw		*90*	*26*
ox, raw		*86*	*24*
ox, stewed		*172*	*49*
pig, raw		*90*	*26*
pig, stewed		*153*	*43*
Kidney, grilled	Sainsbury	106	1 lamb's/2oz 60
Kidney beans (canned drained)	Tesco	121	34
King Cone:	Lyons Maid		
chocolate			per cone 219
Cornish dairy			per cone 208
mint chocolate			per cone 202
strawberry			per cone 191
vanilla			per cone 203
Kipper fillets (frozen)	John West	228	65
	Ross	190	54
	Waitrose	210	57
buttered	Birds Eye	194	55

Product	Brand	Calories per 100g/ 100ml	Calories per oz/ pack/ portion
Kipper fillets			
with butter	Ross	200	57
with butter (box)	St Michael	307	87
Kippered mackerel fillets	Ross	210	60
	St Michael	310	88
Kippers			
baked		*205*	*58*
baked (with bones)		*111*	*31*
Kippers			
(fresh or frozen)	Sainsbury	176	50
(frozen)	Safeway	210	38
	Waitrose	109	31
Loch Fyne	St Michael	368	104
whole Scottish	St Michael	310	88
Kit Kat	Rowntree Mackintosh	505	2-finger pack 110 4-finger pack 230
Knoodles (Knorr) *see under flavours*			
Korma Classic Curry	Homepride	91	383g pack 350
Korma curry mix (as sold)	Colman's	335	95
Kracka Wheat	McVitie		per biscuit 37
Krajana, Polish	Sainsbury	123	35
Krispen:	Lyons		
standard		390	per slice 17
whole rye		375	per slice 16
whole wheat with bran		360	per slice 16

Product	Brand	Calories per 100g/ 100ml	Calories per oz/ pack/ portion
Lager (bottled)		29	8
Lager	Sainsbury	28	½ pint 80
Red Stripe strong	H.P. Bulmer	45	13
Lager and lime	Waitrose	31	9
Lager shandy	Minster	27	8
LAMB			
breast, raw, lean and fat		378	107
roast, lean and fat		410	116
roast, lean only		252	71
chops, grilled	Sainsbury	176	1 chop/6oz 300
			1 chop lean only 125
cutlets, grilled, lean and fat		370	105
grilled, lean and fat (with bone)		244	69
grilled, lean only		222	63
grilled, lean only (with fat and bone)		97	27
raw, lean and fat		386	109
dressed carcase, raw		333	94
fat, average, cooked		616	175
average, raw		671	190
lean, average, raw		162	46
leg	St Michael	240	68
raw, lean and fat		240	68
roast, lean and fat		266	75
roast, lean and fat	Sainsbury	265	1 slice/2oz 150
roast, lean only		191	54
roast, lean only	Sainsbury	194	1 slice/2oz 110

Product	Brand	Calories per 100g/ 100ml	Calories per oz/ pack/ portion
LAMB			
loin chops, grilled, lean and fat		*355*	*101*
grilled, lean and fat (with bone)		*277*	*79*
grilled, lean only		*222*	*63*
grilled, lean only (with fat and bone)		*122*	*35*
raw, lean and fat		*377*	*107*
scrag and neck, raw, lean and fat		*316*	*90*
stewed, lean and fat		*292*	*83*
stewed, lean only		*253*	*72*
stewed, lean only (with fat and bone)		*128*	*36*
shoulder	St Michael	314	89
raw, lean and fat		314	89
roast, lean and fat		316	90
roast, lean and fat	Sainsbury	317	1 slice/2oz 180
roast, lean only		196	56
roast, lean only	Sainsbury	194	1 slice/2oz 110
Lamb grills	St Michael	377	107
	Tiffany's	210	per grill 194
Lamb ragout (Cook in the Pot)	Crosse & Blackwell	389	110
Lamb savouries	Tiffany's	260	per savoury 260
Lamb stuffing	Whitworths	334	95

152

Product	Brand	Calories per 100g/ 100ml	Calories per oz/ pack/ portion
Lancashire cheese	Sainsbury	353	100
	St Michael	380	108
	Tesco	353	100
	Waitrose	423	120
Lard		*891*	*253*
Lard	Armour	930	264
	Safeway	924	262
	Sainsbury	882	1 tbsp/½oz 125
	Tesco	931	264
American	Waitrose	924	262
English refined	Waitrose	924	262
Lasagne	Crosse & Blackwell	112	32
(as sold)	Buitoni	334	95
(frozen)	Birds Eye	123	9oz pack 315
	BHS	104	454g pack 472
minced beef	St Michael	95	27
verdi (as sold)	BHS	343	97
	Buitoni	334	95
Lattice sausage roll with onion	BHS	348	206g pack 718
Laverbread		*52*	*15*
Leek soup *see also Cream of Leek*			
Leek soup (as sold)	Knorr	355	101
Leeks			
boiled		*24*	*7*
raw		*31*	*9*
Leeks, boiled	Sainsbury	25	7
Leeks with cheese sauce	St Michael	127	36

Product	Brand	Calories per 100g/ 100ml	Calories per oz/ pack/ portion
Leicester cheese	Sainsbury	370	105
	St Michael	390	111
	Waitrose	423	120
Lemon and barley squash	Sainsbury	16	½ pint diluted from 4 tbsp 45
Lemon and lime			
(canned)	Safeway	49	14
(mixer)	Safeway	20–30	6–9
Lemon and lime barley water	Robinsons	105	30
Lemon and lime drink	BHS	87	25
	Waitrose	35	10
bittersweet low calorie sparkling (canned)	Hunts	5	1.5
concentrated (as sold)	Idris	93	26
	Quosh	99	28
	Safeway	90	26
concentrated (made up)	Sainsbury	18	½ pint diluted from 4 tbsp 50
Lemon and lime fruit drink	St Michael	35	10
Lemon and lime marmalade	Rose's	260	74
Today's Recipe	Robertson's	180	51
Lemon and lime whole fruit drink	Robinsons	95	27
Lemon and parsley Coat & Cook	Homepride	442	43g pack 190

Product	Brand	Calories per 100g/ 100ml	Calories per oz/ pack/ portion
Lemon and barley drink (undiluted)			
	Quosh	96	27
	Tesco	126	36
Lemon barley water (undiluted)			
	Corona	90	26
	Robinsons	105	30
	Waitrose	142	42
Lemon cheese	Hartley's	295	84
	Moorhouse	295	84
Lemon cordial, low calorie (made up)	PLJ	24	7
Lemon cream filled bar	St Michael	420	119
Lemon cream flan	St Michael	365	103
Lemon creams	Crawford		per biscuit 63
Lemon crispy creams	Tesco	503	143
Lemon crumble creams	Tesco	504	143
Lemon curd, home made starch base		290	82
		283	80
Lemon curd	Gales	290	82
	Moorhouse	285	81
	Robertson's	291	82
	Sainsbury	282	1 tbsp/1oz 80
	Tesco	331	94
	Waitrose	303	86
Lemon curd tarts	Sainsbury		per tart 125
	Waitrose	504	143
Lemon drink	BHS	90	26
	BHS	34	320ml 108
	Waitrose	122	36

155

Product	Brand	Calories per 100g/ 100ml	Calories per oz/ pack/ portion
Lemon drink			
concentrated			
(undiluted)	Kia-Ora	101	29
	Quosh	101	29
	Schweppes	108	31
	Tesco	101	29
concentrated			
2-fold (undiluted)	Suncrush	192	54
low calorie	Chekwate	25	7
	Safeway	3	negl.
	Tesco	21	6
Party (undiluted)	Idris	90	26
whole (undiluted)	Corona	94	27
	Idris	91	26
Lemon drink with lime juice			
canned	Tango	34	9.5
sparkling (bottled)	Tango	37	10
Lemon Jelly Cream	Chivers	370	105
Lemon jelly dessert	Chivers	270	77
(as sold)	Waitrose	258	73
Lemon jelly	Safeway	252	72
marmalade	Waitrose	261	74
Lemon juice	Jif	30	8.5
	Rose's	6	2
	Tesco	7	2
	Waitrose	7	2
fresh		7	*2*
original sharp			
(made up)	PLJ	24	7

Product	Brand	Calories per 100g/ 100ml	Calories per oz/ pack/ portion
Lemon marmalade			
fine shred	Baxters	251	12oz/340g jar 853
Tangy Lemon Shred	Chivers	260	74
Lemon meringue pie		*323*	*92*
Lemon Puffs	Peek Frean	506	per biscuit 67
Lemon Rise and Shine	Kellogg's	313 (dry)	4fl.oz/114ml 47
Lemon sole			
fried		*216*	*61*
fried (with bones)		*171*	*48*
raw		*81*	*23*
steamed		*91*	*26*
steamed (with bones and skin)		*64*	*18*
Lemon sole, fillets	St Michael	77	22
fillets in breadcrumbs	St Michael	120	34
on the bone (frozen)	Waitrose	63	18
Lemon sorbet (2 litre)	Wall's		per pack 1505
Lemon squash (diluted)	Sainsbury	16	½ pint diluted from 4 tbsp 45
(undiluted)	Britvic	96	27
	Idris	111	31
	Safeway	90	26
	Waitrose	122	36
diabetic with glucose (diluted)	Rose's	5	1.5
(diluted)	Sainsbury	25	½ pint diluted from 4 tbsp 70

Product	Brand	Calories per 100g/ 100ml	Calories per oz/ pack/ portion
Lemon torte	Ross	250	71
Lemon water ice	Sainsbury	70	20
Lemon whole fruit drink	Robinsons	95	27
Lemon yogurt	Waitrose	95	27
Lemon/lime	Schweppes	40	11
Lemon/lime drink, concentrated (undiluted)	Kia-Ora	99	28
Lemon/lime yoghurt	Eden Vale	92	26
Lemonade (bottled)		21	6
Lemonade	Barr	33	9.5
	BHS	23	6.5
	Britvic	33	9.5
	Cascade	20	6
	Club	22	113ml 25, 185ml 45
	Idris	24	7
	Minster	20	6
	Safeway	20–30	6–9
	Sainsbury	30	½ pint 85
	Schweppes	27	8
	Tesco	22	6
	Waitrose	35	10
	Zing	40	11
canned	Safeway	39	11
low calorie	Slimsta	4	1
slimline	Schweppes	5	1.5
sparkling	Corona	24	7
	Hunts	24	7
(canned)	Corona	24	7
low calorie	Hunts	4	1

Product	Brand	Calories per 100g/ 100ml	Calories per oz/ pack/ portion
Lemonade and beer shandy, slimline	Schweppes	6	2
Lemonade and cider	Top Deck	38	11
Lemonade shandy	Schweppes	25	7
	Waitrose	24	7
canned	Corona	25	7
	Safeway	53	15
	Top Deck	25	7
Lemons, whole		*15*	*4.5*
Lentil and vegetable casserole	Granose	91	26
Lentil soup		*99*	*28*
Lentil soup			
canned	Baxters	47	15oz/425g can 199
	Heinz	60	17
condensed (undiluted)	Campbell's	94	27
	Granny's	57	16
Lentil with vegetable soup, Scottish	Crosse & Blackwell	45	13
Lentils			
cooked (boiled)		*99*	*28*
cooked (boiled)	Granose	107	30
	Sainsbury	106	1 tbsp/1oz 30
	Whitworths	99	28
masur dahl, cooked		*90*	*26*
raw (dry)		*304*	*86*
raw (dry)	Safeway	297	84
	Sainsbury	317	1 tbsp/1oz 90
	Tesco	297	84

Product	Brand	Calories per 100g/ 100ml	Calories per oz/ pack/ portion
Lentils	Waitrose	296	84
	Whitworths	304	86
Lessen	Farley		per serving (drink + 1 biscuit) 150
Lettuce, raw		*12*	*3.5*
Lettuce, raw	Sainsbury		4 leaves/1oz negl.
Licorice toffees, bag, box or loose	Callard & Bowser, Nuttall	470	per sweet 40
roll		470	per sweet
Light crispbread	St Michael	390	per piece 17
Light madeira cake	Sainsbury	400	¹/₅ cake/1½oz 170
Lightly fruited cake	Sainsbury	326	¹/₆ cake/2oz 185
Lilt	Coca Cola	38	185ml 70, 325ml 140
Lime and lemon crush	Britvic	50	14
Lime curd	Gales	300	85
Lime flavoured cordial (undiluted)	Corona	90	26
	Quosh	90	26
	Schweppes	96	27
Lime Jelly dessert (as sold)	Chivers	265	75
	Waitrose	258	73
Lime juice cordial (diluted)	Sainsbury	18	½ pint diluted from 4 tbsp 50

160

Product	Brand	Calories per 100g/ 100ml	Calories per oz/ pack/ portion
Lime juice cordial			
(undiluted)		*112*	*32*
(undiluted)	Britvic	90	26
	Idris	95	27
	Robinson's	90	26
	Rose's	95	27
	Waitrose	108	32
low calorie	Chekwate	8	2.5
Lime marmalade	Rose's	260	74
Lime squash	Safeway	90	26
Limeade	Idris	23	6.5
	Minster	26	7
	Tesco	20	6
sparkling	Corona	23	6.5
Limeade and lager			
(canned)	Corona	32	9
	Top Deck	32	9
Lincoln biscuits	McVitie		per biscuit 38
	Peek Frean	486	per biscuit 35
	Sainsbury		per biscuit 45
	Tesco	494	140
Lincoln pea soup, thick (5 min.)	Batchelors		per pack 241
Lin-O-Saf margarine	Alfonal	732	208
Lin-O-Saf oil	Alfonal	900	255
Lion Bar	Rowntree Mackintosh	490	per pack 215
Liqueur chocolate assortment	Famous Names	442	125
Liquorice allsorts		*313*	*89*

Product	Brand	Calories per 100g/ 100ml	Calories per oz/ pack/ portion
Liquorice allsorts	Bassett's	367	104
	Sainsbury	300	85
	St Michael	368	104
	Waitrose	317	90
Liquorice comfits	Sainsbury	335	95
Liquorice novelties	Bassett's	314	89
Liquorice sticks	St Michael	389	110
Liquorice toffees *see Licorice*			
Liver			
calf, fried		*254*	*72*
calf, raw		*153*	*43*
chicken, fried		*194*	*55*
chicken, raw		*135*	*38*
lamb, fried		*232*	*66*
lamb, raw		*179*	*51*
ox, raw		*163*	*46*
ox, stewed		*198*	*56*
pig, raw		*154*	*44*
pig, stewed		*189*	*54*
Liver, grilled	Sainsbury	159	thin slice 45
Liver, lamb	St Michael	179	51
Liver and bacon paste	Shippams	195	55
Liver and bacon roll	Crosse & Blackwell	248	70
Liver sausage		*310*	*88*
Liver sausage	Sainsbury	282	80
Belgian	Sainsbury	317	90
coarse	BHS	313	89
Continental	Sainsbury	282	80
smoked German	Sainsbury	335	95
smooth	BHS	376	107

Product	Brand	Calories per 100g/ 100ml	Calories per oz/ pack/ portion
Liver with onion and gravy	Birds Eye		per pack 190
Lobster, boiled (weighed with shell)		119 42	34 12
Lobster bisque	Baxters	42	15oz/425g can 180
	Crosse & Blackwell	38	11
Lobster pâté	Princes	134	38
Lobster soup	Sainsbury	67	½ pint 190
	Waitrose	64	19
Lockets	Mars		per packet 154 per sweet 15
Loganberries			
canned		101	29
raw		17	5
stewed with sugar		54	15
stewed without sugar		16	4.5
Loganberries, canned drained	Tesco	78	22
Lollies	Trebor		per lolly 45
Lollipops	St Michael	385	109
London Grill	Crosse & Blackwell	157	45
Long pie/Long pie with egg	Sainsbury	335	95
Loops (savoury snack)	St Michael	480	136
Low fat spread		366	104
Low fat spread	Safeway	360	103
	Sainsbury	388	1 tbsp/½oz 55

Product	Brand	Calories per 100g/ 100ml	Calories per oz/ pack/ portion
Lucozade		*68*	*19*
Lucozade	Beecham Foods	74	21
Lunch tongue	Sainsbury	300	85
Luncheon meat, canned		*313*	*89*
Lychees			
canned		*68*	*19*
raw		*64*	*18*

Product	Brand	Calories per 100g/ 100ml	Calories per oz/ pack/ portion
McVities wafers	McVitie		per biscuit 90
Macaroni, boiled		*117*	*33*
Macaroni, boiled	Whitworths	117	33
quick, raw	Buitoni	334	95
raw (dry)		*370*	*105*
raw (dry)	BHS	346	98
	James Marshall	320	91
	Sainsbury	388	1 tbsp/½oz 55
	Waitrose	360	102
	Whitworths	370	105
Macaroni beef soup (undiluted)	Granny's	101	29
Macaroni cheese		*174*	*49*
Macaroni cheese	Crosse & Blackwell	102	29
	Heinz	123	35
Macaroni pudding	Sainsbury	96	27
creamed	Ambrosia	106	15½oz can 465
	Safeway	144	45
	Waitrose	130	37
MACKEREL			
canned	Sainsbury	300	85
fillets	BHS	280	79
	Libby	174	49
fillets in oil (drained)	John West	325	92
fillets in tomato sauce	John West	207	92
fried		*188*	*53*
fried (with bones)		*138*	*39*

Product	Brand	Calories per 100g/ 100ml	Calories per oz/ pack/ portion
MACKEREL			
kippered fillets	St Michael	310	88
raw		*223*	*63*
smoked	St Michael	150	43
smoked fillets	Ross	270	77
smoked fillets in oil (drained)	John West	314	89
steaks in natural juice	John West	290	82
steaks in tomato sauce	John West	202	57
Macvita	McVitie		per piece 46
Macvita, New	McVitie		per piece 33
Madeira cake		*393*	*111*
Madeira cake	Sainsbury	400	¹/₅ cake/1½oz 170
	Waitrose	384	109
all butter	St Michael	405	115
butter	BHS	443	126
	Lyons	380	per cake 760
light	Sainsbury	400	¹/₅ cake/1½oz 170
mini	Sainsbury		per cake 80
Madeira Christmas cake, iced top all butter	St Michael	413	117
Madeira cut cake, all butter	St Michael	401	114
Madeira sandwich cake, all butter, iced	St Michael	389	110
Madeira wine sauce (Cooking-in)	Baxters	58	425g can 245

Product	Brand	Calories per 100g/ 100ml	Calories per oz/ pack/ portion
Madelines	Waitrose	247	70
Madras Classic Curry	Homepride	99	383g pack 380
Madras curry (as sold)	Beanfeast	269	per pack 309
Madras Curry (Cook in the Pot)	Crosse & Blackwell	442	125
Madras curry mix (as sold)	Colman's	335	95
Madras curry powder	Whitworths	233	66
Madras hot curry sauce (Cooking-In)	Baxters	72	425g can 307
Maizy oil	Alfonal	900	255
Mallows *see also Coconut, Jamboree, etc*			
Mallows milk or plain coated	Jacobs	420	per biscuit 56
ring	Peek Frean	384	per biscuit 49
Malt bread		*248*	*70*
Malt flavour drink	Cup-a-Time	394	per pack 130
Malt loaf	Sainsbury	282	1 thin slice/ 1oz 80
Malted chocolate	Tesco	390	111
Malted chocolate flavour drink	Cup-a-Time	434	per pack 126
Malted drink	Tesco	398	113
Malted milk (as sold)	Safeway	386	110
	Waitrose	398	113
(made up)	Sainsbury	74	½ pint (3 tsp with half milk/ water) 210
Malted milk bears	Waitrose	465	132

Product	Brand	Calories per 100g/ 100ml	Calories per oz/ pack/ portion
Malted milk biscuits	BHS	488	138
	Sainsbury		per biscuit 35
	Tesco	512	145
Maltesers	Mars		medium pack 180
			per sweet 10
Malty biscuits	Chiltonian		per biscuit 37
	Peek Frean	486	per biscuit 39
Mandarin orange flan filling	Armour	115	33
Mandarin oranges (canned)		*56*	*16*
Mandarin oranges			
canned	BHS	68	19
	Libby	56	16
	Safeway	64	18
	Waitrose	63	18
canned (drained)	Tesco	63	18
canned (inc. syrup)	Sainsbury	66	1 tbsp/1oz 19
canned (segments in natural juice)	John West	30	8.5
canned (segments in syrup)	John West	53	15
Mandarin Royale	St Michael	139	39
Mandarin yoghurt	Waitrose	95	27
Mango chutney	Pan Yan	215	61
Mango chutney, sweet	Crosse & Blackwell	229	65
Mangoes, canned		*77*	*22*
raw		*59*	*17*
Maple and Walnut Jelly Cream	Chivers	370	105

Product	Brand	Calories per 100g/ 100ml	Calories per oz/ pack/ portion
Maple walnut ice cream	Wall's	180	270g pack 485
Marathon:	Mars		
funsize			each 103
single			each 257
Marble cake	Sainsbury	397	1/7 cake/2oz 225
Margarine (all kinds)		*730*	*207*
Margarine	Sainsbury	776	1 tbsp/½oz 110
(all brands)	Van den Berghs	740	210
(all types) all vegetable	Tesco	776	220
(de luxe)	Safeway	740	211
blended (table-tubs) block (cooking and	Safeway	740	211
table)	Safeway	740	211
Gold	St Ivel	375	106
hard	Waitrose	797	226
luxury pure vegetable	Kraft	751	213
(sunflower)	Safeway	740	211
soft	Waitrose	797	226
soft spread	BHS	606	250g pack 1515
sunflower	Kraft	751	213
superfine	Kraft	751	213
supersoft	BHS	606	250g pack 1515
superspread	St Michael	730	207

Product	Brand	Calories per 100g/ 100ml	Calories per oz/ pack/ portion
Margeurita pizza (6 per pack)	St Michael	218	62
Maribo cheese (45 % fat in the dry matter)	Danish	344	98
Marie biscuits	Crawford		per biscuit 31
	Sainsbury		per biscuit 30
	Tesco	440	125
Marmalade see also brand names; Lemon, Orange, etc			
Marmalade		261	74
Marmalade	Sainsbury	265	1 tbsp/1oz 75
coarse cut	Tesco	279	79
jelly	Tesco	279	79
matured	Waitrose	261	74
original thick cut	Robertson's	251	71
thick cut	BHS	260	74
	Safeway	263	75
	Waitrose	261	74
thin cut	BHS	260	74
	Tesco	279	79
	Waitrose	261	74
Marmite		179	51
Marmite	Beecham Foods	217	62
Marrow			
boiled		7	2
raw		16	4.5
Mars Bar		441	125
Mars Bar:	Mars		
funsize			each 107
single			each 328
Marshmallows	BHS	338	96

Product	Brand	Calories per 100g/ 100ml	Calories per oz/ pack/ portion
Marshmallows	Pascall	321	91
	Sainsbury	317	90
	Tesco	310	88
Marvel (as sold)	Cadbury's	345	98
Maryland salad	Eden Vale	156	44
Marzipan (almond paste)		*443*	*126*
Marzipan (almond)	Tesco	412	117
	Whitworths	412	117
Marzipan topped cake, all butter	St Michael	368	104
Matchmakers:	Rowntree Mackintosh		
coffee flavour		485	5 sweets 40
mint flavour		480	5 sweets 40
orange flavour		485	5 sweets 40
Matchmakers, long:	Rowntree Mackintosh		
mint flavour		480	per sweet 20
orange flavour		485	per sweet 20
Matriciana Italian sauce	Homepride		376g pack 285
Matzos		*384*	*109*
Matzos	St Michael	375	per biscuit 80
Mayonnaise		*718*	*204*
Mayonnaise	BHS	750	213
	Hellmann's	325	92
	St Michael	718	204
	Tesco	760	215
low calorie	Slimway Heinz	353	100
sunflower	Kraft	758	215

Product	Brand	Calories per 100g/ 100ml	Calories per oz/ pack/ portion
Mazola corn oil	CPC	900	255
Meat and potato pasty	Sainsbury	309	4oz 350
Meat and potato pie family	Ross	280	79
fresh	Tesco	273	77
Meat and vegetable pie	Kraft	354	113g/4oz pie 400
Meat paste		*173*	*49*
Meat pie *see also Chicken and ham, Minced beef, etc*			
Meat pie	Sainsbury	326	4oz pie 370
Meat pudding	Goblin	200	142g pudding 285
Meatballs	Danish Prime	245	69
	Ross	240	68
in gravy	Campbell's	110	31
in onion gravy	Campbell's	132	37
in tomato sauce	Campbell's	129	37
	Tesco	101	29
with onion and gravy	Tesco	120	34
Meatless savoury cuts	Granose	88	25
Meaux mustard	Colman's	150	42
Mediterranean stir-fry vegetables (fried)	Birds Eye	106	30
Medium curry sauce (Cooking-In)	Baxters	72	425g can 307
Medlars, raw		*42*	*12*
Melba	Birds Eye		per tub 130

Product	Brand	Calories per 100g/100ml	Calories per pack/portion
Melba toast	Buitoni	382	108
Melon, canteloupe			
raw		*24*	*7*
raw (with skin)		*15*	*4.5*
Melon, canteloupe	Sainsbury	18	4oz wedge 20
honeydew	Sainsbury	13	4oz wedge 15
yellow, honeydew			
raw		*21*	*6*
raw (with skin)		*13*	*4*
Melton Mowbray pie,			
5oz	Sainsbury	380	whole 540
9oz	Sainsbury	388	whole 990
16oz	Sainsbury	392	¼ pie/4oz 445
Meringue nests	Sainsbury		per nest 55
	St Michael	380	per nest 61
Meringues		*380*	*108*
Meringues	Waitrose	497	141
Meringues (4 per pack)	St Michael	338	each 118
Merlins Brew	Lyons Maid		each 65
Mexican bean stew	Granose	124	35
Mexican chilli			
(as sold)	Beanfeast	292	per pack 335
Mexicorn (all sizes)	Green Giant	86	24
Milanese sauce	Buitoni	50	14
Mild Burger mustard	Colman's	110	31
Mild curry (as sold)	Beanfeast	282	per pack 324
Mild English mustard	Colman's	185	52
Mild mustard pickle	Baxters	143	291g jar 414
	Heinz	130	33

Product	Brand	Calories per 100g/ 100ml	Calories per oz/ pack/ portion
Milk see also Condensed, Instant, etc			
Milk, cows'			
dried, skimmed		355	101
dried, whole		490	139
fresh, skimmed		33	9.5
fresh, whole		65	18
fresh, whole, Channel Islands		76	22
longlife (UHT treated)		65	18
sterilized		65	18
Milk, cows',			
semi-skimmed	St Michael	52	15
whole	Sainsbury	67	1 tbsp 10, ¼ pint 95
whole (Channel Islands)		77	22
Milk, goats'		71	20
Milk Assorted biscuits: Cadbury's			
barrel		485	137
ring		475	135
sandwich		510	145
triangle		475	135
wafer		530	150
Milk Brazil block	Cadbury's	546	155
Milk caramel wafers	St Michael	493	per biscuit 96
Milk chocolate see also Chocolate			
Milk chocolate and chocolate brazils	BHS	542	154
Milk chocolate and chocolate selection			
(175g)	BHS	519	147
(330g)	BHS	497	141

Product	Brand	Calories per 100g/ 100ml	Calories per oz/ pack/ portion
Milk chocolate bar	BHS	517	147
Milk chocolate bonbons	BHS	499	141
Milk chocolate brazils (175g)	BHS	545	155
Milk chocolate buttons	BHS	508	50g pack 254
	Sainsbury	494	140
Milk chocolate caramel wafers	BHS	472	134
	Sainsbury		each 125
Milk chocolate chums	BHS	198	51g pack 101
Milk chocolate coffee log	BHS	435	40g pack 174
Milk chocolate crisp	BHS	466	42g pack 196
Milk chocolate currant crunch	BHS	485	137
Milk chocolate digestive biscuits	Cadbury's	515	146
	Huntley & Palmers	493	per biscuit 62
	Sainsbury		per biscuit 65
	Tesco	518	147
half coat	St Michael	505	per biscuit 66
Milk chocolate Dundee biscuits	Tesco	483	137
Milk chocolate eggs	Sainsbury	494	140
Milk chocolate fingers	Safeway	516	147
	Sainsbury		per biscuit 70
Milk chocolate flavour bar (cooking)	Tesco	308	87
Milk chocolate fruit and nut	BHS	504	143

Product	Brand	Calories per 100g/ 100ml	Calories per oz/ pack/ portion
Milk chocolate homewheat	McVitie		per biscuit 75
Milk chocolate Jaffa biscuits	Tesco	420	119
Milk chocolate log	BHS		43g pack 200
Milk chocolate mint creams	Tesco	521	148
Milk chocolate orange flavoured fingers	Safeway	515	147
Milk chocolate rings	BHS	500	142
Milk chocolate rum and raisin log	BHS	375	40g pack 150
Milk chocolate sandwich biscuits	BHS	511	145
	Sainsbury		each 140
	Tesco	524	149
Milk chocolate shortcake biscuits	Tesco	513	145
Milk chocolate snack wafers	Sainsbury		per biscuit 100
Milk chocolate sweetmeal	BHS	505	143
	Tesco	504	143
Milk chocolate tea cakes	Tesco	427	121
Milk chocolate toffee rolls	Callard & Bowser	450	per sweet 33
Milk chocolate topped tea biscuits	St Michael	474	per biscuit 72
Milk chocolate wafers	BHS	517	147
	Tesco	420	119
Milk Crunch biscuits	St Michael	487	per biscuit 34

176

Product	Brand	Calories per 100g/ 100ml	Calories per oz/ pack/ portion
Milk Fruit and Nut	Cadbury's	467	132
Milk pudding		*131*	*37*
Milk Tray assortment	Cadbury's	456	129
Milk Tray bar	Cadbury's	484	137
Milk wafer bar	St Michael	510	145
Milk Wholenut	Cadbury's	551	156
Milky Way, funsize	Mars		each 75
single			each 134
Milquick milk powder (made up)	St Ivel	33	1 pint 195
Mince, Scotch	Baxters	110	15¼oz/432g can 476
Mince pies		*435*	*123*
Mince pies	Lyons	392	per pie 194
	Tesco	394	112
puff pastry	St Michael	378	107
short pastry	Sainsbury		per pie 160
	St Michael	375	106
Mince puff pastries	Lyons	464	per pastry 187
Mince Savour	Crosse & Blackwell	326	92
Minceburgers (1¾oz), as sold	Tiffany's	255	per burger 127
Minced beef *see also Beef*			
Minced beef (canned)	St Michael	229	65
Minced beef and onion (canned)	Batchelors		per can 467
	Sainsbury	141	7½oz can 300
	Tesco	163	46
Minced beef and onion pie (142g/5oz)	Kraft		per pie 370

Product	Brand	Calories per 100g/ 100ml	Calories per oz/ pack/ portion
Minced beef and onion pie			
(4½oz oval, baked)	Tiffany's	260	per pie 332
(5oz round, baked)	Tiffany's	250	per pie 355
(1lb, baked)	Tiffany's	250	¼ pie 280
Minced beef and veg. ready meal	Ross	80	23
Minced beef and veg. pie, Value	Birds Eye		pie for 1 410 pie for 2–3 1070
Minced beef and veg. stew	Campbell's	138	39
Minced beef lasagne	St Michael	95	27
Minced beef loaf	Armour	216	61
Minced beef pancakes	Birds Eye		each, shallow fried 130
Minced beef pie	Sainsbury	292	¼ pie/3¾oz 310
canned	Tesco	364	103
large	BHS	329	93
	St Michael	262	74
rich pastry	St Michael	336	95
small	BHS	283	per pie 399
	St Michael	311	88
top crust	St Michael	282	80
Minced beef pie filling	Tesco	124	35
Minced beef roll	St Michael	324	92
baked	BHS	296	342g pack 1012
Minced beef with veg. in gravy	Birds Eye		per pack 150

Product	Brand	Calories per 100g/ 100ml	Calories per oz/ pack/ portion
Minced steak and gravy (canned)	Sainsbury	159	15oz can 675
Minced steak and onion pie filling	Fray Bentos	120	34
Minced steak and vegetables	Campbell's	138	39
Mincemeat		*235*	*67*
Mincemeat	Hartley's	295	84
	Robertson's	266	75
	Safeway	300	85
	Sainsbury	265	1tbsp/1oz 75
	Tesco	129	37
	Waitrose	130	37
with brandy	BHS	294	83
Minestrone soup canned	Granose	28	8
	Baxters	34	15oz/425g can 145
	Crosse & Blackwell	48	14
	Heinz Big Soups	57	16
	Heinz Ready to Serve	43	12
	Sainsbury	60	½ pint 170
dried		*298*	*84*
(as served)		*23*	*65*
dried (as sold)	5-Minute		per pack 153
	Knorr	343	97
	Tesco	362	103
dried (made up)	Chef Box	28	8

Product	Brand	Calories per 100g/ 100ml	Calories per oz/ pack/ portion
Minestrone soup			
dried (made up)	Maggi		
	Quick Cook	34	9.5
	Sainsbury	60	21
with croûtons	Cup-a-Soup		
	Special	292	per portion 70
Mini bricks	Lyons Maid		each 57
Mini choc	Wall's		each 45
Mini fruit	Wall's		each 30
Mini jellies	Sainsbury	317	90
Mini madeira cakes	Sainsbury		per cake 80
Mini milk (strawberry or vanilla)	Wall's		each 35
Mini rolls, chocolate covered	Sainsbury		per roll 145
Mini sticks:	St Michael		
hazelnut		550	156
mint		477	135
mocca		552	156
Mini Wheats	Sainsbury	335	2tbsp/1oz 95
Mini wine gums	St Michael	342	97
Minstrels	Mars		std. pack 218 per sweet 14.
Mint, fresh garden	Colman's	25	7
rubbed	Tesco	300	85
Mint allsorts	Sainsbury	370	105
Mint chocolate bonbons	Parkinsons	404	114
Mint choc chip, Soft Scoop (2 litre)	Wall's		per pack 2300

Product	Brand	Calories per 100g/ 100ml	Calories per oz/ pack/ portion
Mint choc croccante italiano (544g/1 litre)	Wall's	225	per pack 1225
Mint chocolate dessert	Sainsbury		per tub 215
Mint chocolates	Callard & Bowser	420	per sweet 29
Mint Creams (carton)	Clarnico		per pack 763 per sweet 30
Mint creams, milk chocolate	Tesco	521	148
Mint Crisps	Elizabeth Shaw	443	125
Mint humbugs	Sainsbury	370	105
Mint imperials	BHS	372	40g pack 149
	Sainsbury	335	95
	St Michael	370	105
Mint jelly	Baxters	259	185g jar 642
	Colman's	340	96
	Crosse & Blackwell	259	73
	Sainsbury	106	1tbsp/1oz 30
Mint lumps	Parkinsons	381	108
Mint sauce	HP Foods	85	24
	O.K.	50	14
	Safeway	25	7
	Sainsbury	141	1tbsp/1oz 40
	Tesco	100	28
concentrated garden	Baxters	150	160g jar 341
	Pan Yan	45	13
ready to serve	Baxters	150	145g jar 341

Product	Brand	Calories per 100g/ 100ml	Calories per oz/ pack/ portion
Mint sundaes	St Michael	538	per biscuit 87
Mint thins	Parkinsons	378	107
Mint toffees, bag, box or loose	Callard & Bowser, Nuttall	470	per sweet 40
roll	Callard & Bowser, Nuttall	470	per sweet 23
Mint Toffo	Rowntree Mackintosh	455	per sweet 20
Minted peas *see Peas*			
Mintoes	St Michael	410	116
bag, box or loose	Callard & Bowser, Nuttall	380	per sweet 27
stick pack		380	per sweet 16
Mintola	Rowntree Mackintosh	440	per sweet 25
Mints, old fashioned	Parkinsons	378	107
Mr. Chew (all flavours)		381	108
Mr. Men (all types)	Lyons Maid		each 25
Mivvi, strawberry	Lyons Maid		each 78
Mixed dried fruit	Safeway	247	70
	Tesco	247	70
	Waitrose	247	70
	Whitworths	245	69
Mixed fruit jam	Moorhouse	260	74
	Safeway	270	76
	Tesco	279	79
Mixed fruit pickle	Baxters	173	305g jar 526

Product	Brand	Calories per 100g/100ml	Calories per oz/pack/portion
Mixed fruit pudding	Heinz	307	87
	Sainsbury	349	per can 1040
Mixed fruit sponge pudding	Goblin		297g pack 800
Mixed grain bread	St Michael	225	64
Mixed grain rolls	St Michael	224	64
Mixed herbs, rubbed	Tesco	300	85
Mixed Nut Assortment	Cadbury's	547	155
Mixed nuts	St Michael	582	165
chopped	Sainsbury	529	150
	Whitworths	564	160
roasted	Tesco	750	213
salted	Sun-Pat	605	172
Mixed peel	Safeway	282	80
	Whitworths	244	69
cut	Tesco	243	69
	Waitrose	261	74
Mixed peppers, dried	Batchelors	295	46g pack 136
	Tesco	205	58
Mixed pickles	Crosse & Blackwell	2	
	Epicure	4	1
	Haywards	9	2.5
sweet	Crosse & Blackwell	131	37
Mixed salad	St Michael	17	5
in French dressing	Tesco	73	21
Mixed spice, ground	Tesco	300	85
	Whitworths	253	72
Mixed vegetable soup	Safeway	45	12

183

Product	Brand	Calories per 100g/ 100ml	Calories per oz/ pack/ portion
Mixed vegetables			
canned	Hartley's	55	16
canned drained	Tesco	46	13
dried	Batchelors	273	53g jar 145
	Sainsbury	282	1tbsp/1oz 80
(cooked)		106	1tbsp/1oz 30
	Tesco	325	92
dried, big value	Batchelors	270	88g pack 238
farmhouse	Ross	40	11
frozen	Ross	55	16
frozen or canned and drained	Sainsbury	35	1tbsp/1oz 10
original	Birds Eye	53	15
special (frozen)	Tesco	68	19
stewpack	Ross	25	7
summer (canned, drained)	Tesco	321	91
supreme (frozen)	BHS	47	454g pack 213
Montego, coconut, ginger or orange flavour	Rowntree Mackintosh	515	146
Morello cherry Viennese	Tiffany's Upper Crust	260	¼ dessert 375
Mornay Master Sauce (as sold)	Colman's	370	105
Morning Coffee biscuits	Peek Frean	440	per biscuit 22
	Pennywise		per biscuit 21
	Sainsbury		per biscuit 20
	Tesco	476	135
	Waitrose	455	129

Product	Brand	Calories per 100g/ 100ml	Calories per oz/ pack/ portion
Mortadella	BHS	219	62
Italian	Sainsbury	353	100
Moussaka		*195*	*55*
Mousse	Sainsbury		per tub 145
Muesli		*368*	*104*
Muesli	Granose	321	91
	Prewetts	359	102
bran	Prewetts	308	87
Country	Jordans	352	100
honey	Prewetts	366	104
Muesli base	Jordans	345	98
	Prewetts	370	105
Muesli biscuits	Allinson	486	138
Muesli cookies	St Michael	476	per biscuit 79
Muesli Deluxe	Prewetts	390	111
Muesli fruit bar	Prewetts	303	86
Muesli yogurt/yoghurt	Country Prize	96	27
	St Michael	112	32
Mulberries, raw		*36*	*10*
Mulligatawny soup	Heinz	59	17
Munch Bunch:	Eden Vale		
banana		102	29
blackberry		105	30
orange		98	28
strawberry		105	30
Munchies	Rowntree Mackintosh	505	per sweet 25
Munchmallows	McVitie		per biscuit 73
Murray Blue Mints	Pascall	377	107

Product	Brand	Calories per 100g/ 100ml	Calories per oz/ pack/ portion
Murray Buttermints	Pascall	409	116
Murray Fruits	Pascall	378	107
Murraymints	Pascall	410	116
Muscovado sugar	Tesco	383	109
Museli	BHS	374	106
Museli, wholewheat	Tesco	377	107
Museli biscuits	BHS	470	133
Mushroom and bacon Toast Topper	Heinz	123	35
Mushroom Omelette Mate	Campbell's	63	18
Mushroom Pasta Menu	Crosse & Blackwell	104	29
Mushroom sauce mix (as sold)	Colman's	335	95
Mushroom soup *see also Cream of mushroom*			
Mushroom soup			
canned	Sainsbury	53	½ pint 150
condensed (diluted)	Campbell's Bumper Harvest	49	14
dried (as sold)	Cup-a-Soup	460	portion 115
	Tesco	362	103
dried (made up)	Chef Box Maggi	28	8
	Quick Cook	32	9
	Sainsbury	21	½ pint 60
Country (as sold)	Knorr	384	109
thick	Cup-a-Soup Special	372	per portion 108

Product	Brand	Calories per 100g/ 100ml	Calories per oz/ pack/ portion
Mushrooms			
fried		210	60
raw		13	3.5
Mushrooms, canned			
drained (all packs)	Tesco	31	9
dried	Tesco	325	92
	Whitworths	138	39
fresh, frozen or			
canned and drained	Sainsbury		2tbsp/1oz negl.
fried	Sainsbury	229	1tbsp/1oz 65
Mushy peas			
(canned drained)	Tesco	243	69
Mussels			
boiled		87	25
boiled (weighed			
with shells)		26	7.5
raw		66	19
Mustard and cress,			
raw		10	3
Mustard piccalilli	Epicure	23	6.5
Mustard powder		452	128
Mustard powder	Colman's	480	136
Mustard relish, mild	Tesco	128	36
Mutton stock cubes	Knorr	298	9.5g cube 28
Mycella cheese	Sainsbury	388	110

Product	Brand	Calories per 100g/ 100ml	Calories per oz/ pack/ portion
Napolitan sauce	Buitoni	27	7.5
Prego, undiluted	Campbell's	93	26
Natural Dry Cider	Taunton	34	1 pint 200
Natural wheels	BHS	505	143
Natural yogurt/yoghurt		52	15
Natural yogurt/yoghurt	BHS	60	per pack 90
	Eden Vale	70	20
	St Ivel	60	17
	Waitrose	56	16
(unsweetened)	Safeway	36	10
	Sainsbury	46	tub/$\frac{1}{4}$ pint 65
	St Michael	69	20
Natural yogurt and grapefruit	Eden Vale	86	24
Natural yogurt and honey	Eden Vale	90	26
Navarine of lamb Casserole Mix (as sold)	Colman's	325	92
Neapolitan cutting brick	Lyons Maid		per pack 834
Neapolitan Gaiety family brick	Lyons Maid		per pack 397
Neapolitan ice cream	St Michael	177	50
	Tesco	222	63
	Tudor	180	51
	Wall's	178	242g pack 430
sliceable			
(525g/1 litre)	Wall's	178	per pack 935
soft scoop (2 litres)	Wall's		per pack 1875

Product	Brand	Calories per 100g/ 100ml	Calories per oz/ pack/ portion
Neapolitan Supermousse	Birds Eye		per tub 155
Neapolitan wafers	Peek Frean	490	per biscuit 37
Nectarines, raw		50	14
(with stones)		46	13
New England soup	Frank Cooper	48	15oz can 210
New potatoes	Hartley's	70	20
Nibblers corn (frozen)	Green Giant	88	25
Niblets corn (canned or frozen)	Green Giant	83	24
Nice biscuits	Jacobs	456	per biscuit 45
	Peek Frean	445	per biscuit 44
	Sainsbury		per biscuit 35
	St Michael	462	per biscuit 43
	Tesco	494	140
	Waitrose	405	115
finger	Pennywise		per biscuit 30
99 Flake	Cadbury's	525	149
Noodle Doodles	Heinz	63	18
Noodles (as sold)	Buitoni	334	95
Noodles, 2-minute:	Crosse & Blackwell		
beef flavour		127	36
chicken flavour		124	35
Norfolk style veg. with chicken	Knorr Hot Pots	374	45g pack 168
Norwegian blue cheese	Sainsbury	353	100

Product	Brand	Calories per 100g/ 100ml	Calories per oz/ pack/ portion
Number 7 cider (bottled)	H.P. Bulmer	35	10
Nut brittle	Barker & Dobson	428	121
Nutbrawn	Granose	212	60
Nutloaf	Granose	176	50
Nutmeg, ground	Tesco	450	128
	Whitworths	273	77
Nuts *see Brazil, etc; also Mixed*			
Nuts and raisins	Whitworths	462	131
Nuttolene	Granose	298	84
Nutty bar	Rowntree Mackintosh	500	per pack 255
Nutty toffee puffs	St Michael	439	124

Product	Brand	Calories per 100g/100ml	Calories per oz/pack/portion
Oat Krunchies	Quaker Oats	380	108
Oatcake, bran	Allinson	419	119
Oatcakes		441	*125*
Oatcakes	Paterson's	425	120
Oatflake and apple cookies	St Michael	458	per biscuit 76
Oatmeal (raw)		*401*	*114*
Oatmeal	Prewetts	405	115
	Sainsbury	388	1 tbsp/½oz 55
	Whitworths	401	114
Oatmeal biscuits	Allinson	492	139
Oatmeal Crunch biscuits	Sainsbury		per biscuit 30
Oil *see also Vegetable, etc*			
Oil	Sainsbury	882	1 tbsp/½oz 125
Oil-free French dressing	Waistline	13	3.5
Okra, raw		17	5
Old English bread	St Michael	241	68
Old English rolls	St Michael	278	79
Old English toffee	Barker & Dobson	430	122
Olde English Georgian marmalade	Chivers	260	74
Thick cut	Chivers	265	75
Olive oil	Alfonal	930	264
	Crosse & Blackwell	900	255
	Safeway	900	255

Product	Brand	Calories per 100g/ 100ml	Calories per oz/ pack/ portion
Olive oil	Tesco	932	264
	Waitrose	930	264
Olives			
stuffed	Tesco	160	45
stuffed Manzanilla	Crosse & Blackwell	45	13
in brine		103	29
(with stones)		82	23
Omelette Mate *see under flavours*			
Onion, big value dried	Batchelors	314	88g pack 276
Onion, potato and cheese flan	Sainsbury	282	¼ flan/3oz 240
Onion, sliced dried	Batchelors	315	53g pack 167
	Tesco	296	84
	Whitworths	296	84
Onion and parsley Salad Days	Knorr	295	6g pack 18
Onion and pepper Pasta Menu	Crosse & Blackwell	119	34
Onion relish	Crosse & Blackwell	135	38
	Tesco	135	38
Onion ringers	Ross	230	65
Onion rings	Tesco	130	37
(savoury snack)	Safeway	483	138
	Sainsbury	520	147
Onion salt	Tesco	100	28
Onion sauce		99	28
Onion sauce mix (as sold)	Colman's	235	67

Product	Brand	Calories per 100g/ 100ml	Calories per oz/ pack/ portion
Onion sauce mix	Knorr	353	100
(made up)	Chef Box	85	24
	Sainsbury	53	1 tbsp/½oz 15
Onion savoury mash	Yeoman	371	per portion made up 69
Onion soup condensed (undiluted)	Campbell's	61	17
dried (as sold)	Cup-a-Soup	448	portion 112
	Knorr Quick Soups	440	125
dried (made up)	Sainsbury	21	½ pint 60
thick (dried, made up)	Chef Box	29	8
Onion spread, low calorie	Waistline	84	24
Onions, boiled		13	4
fried		345	98
raw		23	6.5
spring, raw		35	10
Onions, chopped (frozen)	Waitrose	25	7
fresh or frozen	Sainsbury	18	1 tbsp/1oz 5
fried	Sainsbury	317	1 tbsp/1oz 90
pickled	BHS	14	4
	Epicure	14	4
	Haywards	16	4.5
	Safeway	23	6.5
	Tesco	18	5
pickled silverskins	Epicure	17	5
	Haywards	20	6

Product	Brand	Calories per 100g/ 100ml	Calories per oz/ pack/ portion
Onions, pickled sweet	Epicure	25	7
	Haywards	25	7
	Tesco	28	8
pickled white	Crosse & Blackwell	2	
Onions and white sauce	Birds Eye	141	5oz pack 200
Opals	Mars		sm packet 125 per sweet 18
Orange, lemon and pineapple drink	Robinsons	95	27
Orange and apple whole fruit drink	Robinsons	95	27
Orange and grapefruit drink (undiluted)	Quosh	99	28
Orange and lemon cup cakes	Lyons	332	per cake 129
	Waitrose	688	195
Orange and lemon drink (undiluted)	Quosh	105	30
Orange and lemon mousse	Waitrose	92	26
Orange and lemon slices	Barker & Dobson	320	91
	Waitrose	328	93
Orange and pineapple drink (undiluted)	Kia-Ora	105	30
	Quosh	98	28
Orange barley water	Robinsons	110	31
Orange 'C'			
reduced calories	Libby	31	9
sweetened	Libby	51	14

Product	Brand	Calories per 100g/ 100ml	Calories per oz/ pack/ portion
Orange chocolates	Callard & Bowser, Nuttall	410	per sweet 28
Orange cream filled bar	St Michael	420	119
Orange creams	Cadbury's	520	147
Orange creams (biscuits)	Peek Frean	489	per biscuit 58
	Pennywise		per biscuit 64
	Tesco	487	138
Orange crisps	St Michael	517	per biscuit 27
Orange crush	Britvic	50	14
	Club	57	185ml 105
	Slimsta	5	1.5
Orange curd	Gales	300	85
Orange drink	BHS	90	26
	BHS	41	320ml 131
	Cresta	28	8
	Waitrose	132	39
	Zing	51	14
bittersweet low calorie sparkling (canned)	Hunts	5	1.5
canned	Safeway	47	13
concentrated (undiluted)		*107*	*30*
concentrated (undiluted)	Kia-Ora	97	27
	Quosh	106	30
	Tesco	126	36
concentrated 2-fold (undiluted)	Suncrush	202	57
low calorie	Chekwate	25	7

195

Product	Brand	Calories per 100g/ 100ml	Calories per oz/ pack/ portion
Orange drink,	Club	3	185ml 5
low calorie	Safeway	11	3
	Tesco	24	7
Party (undiluted)	Idris	99	28
Slimline sparkling	Schweppes	5	1.5
sparkling	Schweppes	30	8.5
	Tango	46	13
	Waitrose	34	10
sparkling (canned)	Hunts	40	11
	Tango	46	13
whole (undiluted)	Corona	105	30
	Idris	95	27
Orange Fruitie	Wall's		each 60
Orange jelly dessert	Chivers	280	79
(as sold)	Waitrose	258	73
Orange jelly marmalade	Waitrose	261	74
Orange juice	Britvic	46	13
	Heinz	61	17
	Prewetts	44	12
	Safeway	38	11
	Schweppes	56	16
	Waitrose	37	11
canned sweetened		51	14
canned unsweetened		33	9.5
fresh		38	11
fresh	BHS	40	11
frozen concentrate	Sainsbury	141	1 tbsp/1oz 40
	St Michael	160	45
natural	Tesco	42	12
sweetened	Club	53	113ml 60

Product	Brand	Calories per 100g/ 100ml	Calories per oz/ pack/ portion
Orange juice,	Hunts	52	15
sweetened	Libby	51	14
	Sainsbury	46	¼ pint 65
UHT	Tesco	49	14
	BHS	43	12
unsweetened	Club	44	113ml 50
	Libby	33	9.5
	Sainsbury	39	¼ pint 55
	Schweppes	48	14
Orange Maid	Lyons Maid		each 49
Orange marmalade	Hartley's	230	65
	Safeway	263	75
fine shred	Baxters	251	340g jar 853
medium cut,			
Today's Recipe	Robertson's	180	51
Scotch	Baxters	260	12oz/340g jar 884
Select	Rose's	260	74
Seville	Waitrose	258	74
Tangy Orange			
Shred	Chivers	260	74
Orange Munch Bunch	Eden Vale	98	28
Orange Rise and Shine	Kellogg's	327 (dry)	4fl.oz/114ml 49
Orange squash			½ pint diluted
(diluted)	Sainsbury	16	from 4 tbsp 45
(undiluted)	Britvic	108	31
	Idris	128	36
	Safeway	100	28
	Schweppes	111	31
	Waitrose	132	39

Product	Brand	Calories per 100g/ 100ml	Calories per oz/ pack/ portion
Orange squash			
diabetic (undiluted)	Rose's	17	5
whole orange (diluted)	Sainsbury	23	½ pint diluted from 4 tbsp 65
Orange whip	St Michael	161	46
Orange whole fruit drink	Robinsons	95	27
Orange yogurt	Ski	93	26
Orangeade	Minster	23	7
	Tesco	18	5
(bottled)	Idris	26	7.5
sparkling (bottled)	Corona	26	7.5
Orange/lemon slices	BHS	300	85
Oranges			
raw		*35*	*10*
raw (with peel and pips)		*26*	*7.5*
Oranges	Sainsbury	28	1 med./5oz 40
Original Crunchy:	Jordans		
bar		464	132
cereal, plain		433	123
cereal with bran and apple		410	116
cereal with honey, almonds and raisins		426	121
Original pickle	Pan Yan	140	40
Original tomato soup (as sold)	Knorr	349	99
Original low fat spread	Van den Berghs	370	105

198

Product	Brand	Calories per 100g/ 100ml	Calories per oz/ pack/ portion
Ovaltine		378	107
Ovaltine	Wander	378	15g/3 heaped tsp 57
chocolate flavoured		393	15g/3 heaped tsp 59
milk chocolate		505	50g square 36 100g square 31
Oven chips *see Chips*			
Oven crunches (as sold)	Ross	150	45
Oven Stars:	Birds Eye		
baked or grilled		229	65
fried		300	85
Ox liver *see Liver*			
Ox tongue	BHS	210	60
sliced	St Michael	170	48
Oxford coarse cut marmalade	Frank Cooper	263	75
Oxo beef drink	Brooke Bond Oxo	100	28
Oxo cubes		229	65
Oxo cubes:	Brooke		
chicken	Bond Oxo	210	60
red		270	76
Oxtail, raw		171	48
stewed		243	69
stewed (with bones)		92	26
Oxtail and vegetable soup	Crosse & Blackwell	38	11
Oxtail soup, canned		44	12

Product	Brand	Calories per 100g/ 100ml	Calories per oz/ pack/ portion
Oxtail soup			
canned	Baxters	44	15oz/425g can 185
	BHS	43	12
	Crosse & Blackwell	49	14
	Heinz	48	14
	St Michael	44	12
	Tesco	54	15
	Waitrose	31	9
condensed (undiluted)	Campbell's Bumper Harvest	47	13
	Campbell's Condensed	82	23
dried		*356*	*101*
(as served)		*27*	*7.5*
dried (as sold)	Cup-a-Soup 5-Minute	366	per portion 77 per pack 159
	Knorr	347	98
	Knorr Quick Soups	354	100
	Tesco	330	94
dried (made up)	Chef Box Maggi	29	8
	Quick Cook	30	8.5
	Sainsbury	21	½ pint 60
low calorie	Heinz	21	6
	Waistline	23	6.5
Oysters, raw		*51*	*14*
(with shells)		*6*	*2*

Product	Brand	Calories per 100g/ 100ml	Calories per oz/ pack/ portion
Pacers	Mars		per packet 215
			per sweet 18
Paella	Crosse & Blackwell	175	50
	Vesta	373	per pack 635
(as sold)	Beanfeast	309	per pack 355
Pale ale	Sainsbury	30	½ pint 85
bottled		32	9
Pancake rolls, crispy	Birds Eye		per roll, fried 105
Pancakes		307	87
Scotch		283	80
Pancakes, Scotch	Sainsbury		per pancake 70
	St Michael	304	86
Paprika and oregano Salad Days	Knorr	281	6g pack 17
Parkin cut cake	St Michael	329	93
Parma ham, sliced	St Michael	300	85
Parmesan cheese	Buitoni	498	141
	Kraft	420	119
	Sainsbury	388	110
	Tesco	410	116
Parsley, raw		21	6
Parsley, rubbed	Tesco	300	85
Parsley and chives Salad Days	Knorr	293	6g pack 18
Parsley and thyme stuffing	Whitworths	355	101

Product	Brand	Calories per 100g/ 100ml	Calories per oz/ pack/ portion
Parsley sauce mix			
(as sold)	Colman's	360	102
	Knorr	360	102
(made up)	Chef Box	105	30
	Sainsbury	53	1tbsp/½oz 15
Parsnips			
boiled		*56*	*16*
raw		*49*	*14*
Parsnips	Sainsbury	53	½in. slice/ 1oz 15
Partridge, roast		*212*	*60*
(with bone)		*127*	*36*
Party biscuits	Sainsbury		per biscuit 30
Party rings	BHS	449	127
	Safeway	447	128
Passionfruit, raw		*34*	*9.5*
(with skin)		*14*	*4*
Pasta	James Marshall	320	91 dry
	Quaker Oats	364	103
	Tesco	360	102
Pasta Menu (Crosse & Blackwell) *see under flavours*			
Pasta salad	St Michael	290	82
Pasta shells/twists	Buitoni	334	95 dry
Pasties *see Beef and mushroom, etc*			
Pastilles		*253*	*72*
Pastry			
choux, cooked		*330*	*94*
choux, raw		*214*	*61*

Product	Brand	Calories per 100g/ 100ml	Calories per oz/ pack/ portion
Pastry			
flaky, cooked		565	160
flaky, raw		427	121
shortcrust, cooked		527	149
shortcrust, raw		455	129
Pastry, frozen	Birds Eye		
puff		423	120
puff sheets			per sheet 360
shortcrust		441	125
Pâté			
country style	St Michael	300	85
farmhouse	St Michael	300	85
Patent Barley	Robinsons	365	103
Paw paw, canned		65	18
Pea and ham soup			
canned	Baxters	53	15oz/425g can 226
	Heinz	66	19
condensed	Campbell's		
(undiluted)	Condensed	134	38
	Campbell's		
	Main-Course	82	23
dried (as sold)	Tesco	386	109
Pea soup, thick			
(dried, made up)	Chef Box	26	7.5
Pea with ham soup			
dried (as sold)	Knorr	347	98
dried (made up)	Chef Box	29	8
	Maggi		
	Quick Cook	31	9

Product	Brand	Calories per 100g/ 100ml	Calories per oz/ pack/ portion
Peach and cream mousse	Waitrose	120	34
Peach blancmange (as sold)	Brown & Polson	328	33g pack 108
Peach jam	Hartley's	235	67
Peach melba	St Michael	113	32
Peach melba cutting brick	Lyons Maid		per pack 925
Peach melba yogurt/ yoghurt	BHS	79	150g pack 119
	St Michael	101	29
	Ski	91	26
Peach Sundae Best	St Ivel	180	51
Peach yogurt	Ski	96	27
Peaches, canned		87	25
Peaches, canned	BHS	78	22
	Libby	69	20
	Safeway	76	19
	Sainsbury		2 halves + 1 tbsp syrup 7
(drained)	Tesco	78	22
(halves or slices)	Waitrose	92	26
(slices in fruit juice)	John West	45	13
(slices in syrup)	John West	67	19
Peaches, dried			
raw		212	60
stewed with sugar		93	26
stewed without sugar		79	22
Peaches, fresh, raw		37	10
(with stones)		32	9
Peaches, fresh, raw	Sainsbury	31	1 × 4oz 35

204

Product	Brand	Calories per 100g/ 100ml	Calories per oz/ pack/ portion
Peanut biscuits	Allinson	488	138
Peanut butter	Granose	586	166
	Prewetts	570	162
	Sainsbury	634	1 tbsp/½oz 90
crunchy or smooth	Gales	600	170
	Safeway	600	170
	Sun-Pat	585	166
	Tesco	618	175
smooth		*623*	*177*
Peanut fingers	St Michael	525	149
Peanut fudge	Callard & Bowser, Nuttall	440	per bar 240
Peanut kernels	Whitworths	570	162
Peanuts	St Michael	593	168
dry roasted	BHS	544	154
	St Michael	544	154
fresh		*570*	*162*
(with shells)		*394*	*112*
roasted	Tesco	670	190
salted		*570*	*162*
salted	BHS	570	162
	Sainsbury	600	170
	Sun-Pat	600	170
Peanuts and raisins	St Michael	400	113
	Sun-Pat	480	136
Pear yogurt	Ski	95	27
Pearl barley *see* Barley			
Pears, canned		*77*	*22*
Pears, canned	Safeway	65	18
(all shapes, drained)	Tesco	67	19

Product	Brand	Calories per 100g/ 100ml	Calories per oz/ pack/ portion
Pears, canned			
(halves)	BHS	76	22
	Libby	69	20
	Sainsbury		2 halves + 1 tbs syrup 75
(halves or slices)	Waitrose	77	22
halves in syrup)	John West	74	21
(quarters in juice)	John West	39	11
Pears, cooking			
raw		*36*	*10*
stewed with sugar		*65*	*18*
stewed without sugar		*30*	*8.5*
Pears, eating		*41*	*12*
(with skin and core)		*29*	*8*
Pears, fresh	Sainsbury	26	1×4oz 30
Peas, canned garden		*47*	*13*
Peas, canned garden	BHS	44	12
	Hartley's	65	18
	Safeway	50	14
	Waitrose	49	14
(drained)	Tesco	60	17
Peas, canned marrowfat	Waitrose	95	27
(drained)	Tesco	78	22
Peas, canned mushy	Batchelors	81	23
(drained)	Tesco	243	69
Peas, canned processed		*80*	*23*
Peas, canned processed	Batchelors	63	19
	Hartley's	110	31
(drained)	Tesco	78	22

Product	Brand	Calories per 100g/ 100ml	Calories per oz/ pack/ portion
Peas, chick			
channa dahl		97	27
cooked, dahl		144	41
raw		320	91
Peas, dried			
boiled		103	29
raw		286	81
Peas, dried	Batchelors	282	258g pack 729
	Surprise		125g pack 320
			62g pack 178
			40g pack 109
(as sold)	Sainsbury	300	85
	Waitrose	275	78
	Whitworths	286	81
(cooked)	Sainsbury	106	30
	Whitworths	103	29
garden	Tesco	270	77
marrowfat	Tesco	414	117
Peas, fresh, boiled		52	15
raw		67	19
Peas, fresh, frozen or canned and drained	Sainsbury	53	1 tbsp/1oz 15
Peas, frozen, boiled		41	12
raw		53	15
Peas, frozen	Birds Eye	53	15
	Ross	80	23
	Tesco	70	20
	Waitrose	63	18
(cooked)	Safeway	64	18
(petits pois)	St Michael	53	15
minted	BHS	53	340g pack 181
	Tesco	70	20

Product	Brand	Calories per 100g/ 100ml	Calories per oz/ pack/ portion
Peas, quick dried	Waitrose	303	86
Peas, quick soak	Batchelors	283	254g pack 719
Peas, split dried			
boiled		*118*	*33*
raw		*310*	*88*
Peas, split dried			
(cooked)	Sainsbury	106	1 tbsp/1oz 30
(raw)	Safeway	303	86
	Sainsbury	300	1 tbsp/1oz 85
	Waitrose	303	86
Peas, sweetcorn and peppers	Birds Eye	53	15
Peas, yellow split dried			
raw	Tesco	314	89
boiled	Whitworths	310	88
Peas and baby carrots	Birds Eye	35	10
Peas and carrots, dried			
raw	Sainsbury	265	1 tbsp/1oz 75
cooked		88	25
Pease pudding (canned)	Tesco	90	26
Penguin	McVitie		per biscuit 140
Pennywise biscuits *see Jam Rings, etc*			
Peperonata	Buitoni	50	14
Pepper		*308*	*87*
Peppermint cordial			
(undiluted)	Britvic	90	26
	Club	22	113ml 25
	Idris	120	34
non-alcoholic			
(undiluted)	Schweppes	104	29

208

Product	Brand	Calories per 100g/ 100ml	Calories per oz/ pack/ portion
Peppermint cream	Cadbury's	420	119
Peppermints		*392*	*111*
<u>Peppers, dried</u>	Whitworths	205	58
Peppers, green			
boiled		*14*	*4*
raw		*15*	*4.5*
Pepsi Cola	Schweppes	42	12
Diet	Schweppes	0.25	
Perrier mineral water	H.P. Bulmer	nil	
Petite beurre biscuits	Sainsbury		per biscuit 30
Petits pois, frozen	BHS	53	340g pack 180
	St Michael	53	15
(canned drained)	Tesco	52	15
Pheasant, roast		*213*	*60*
(with bone)		*134*	*38*
Pheasant consommé	Baxters	11.5	15oz/425g can 49
Pheasant soup *see Cream of pheasant*			
Philadelphia cheese	Kraft	317	90
Phosferine Tonic Wine	Beecham Foods	142	40
Piccalilli		*33*	*9.5*
Piccalilli			
	BHS	50	14
	Haywards	29	8
	Happy Farm	33	9.5
	Heinz	73	21
	Pan Yan	85	24
	Tesco	56	16
diced	Crosse & Blackwell	42	12

Product	Brand	Calories per 100g/ 100ml	Calories per oz/ pack/ portion
Piccalilli			
diced sweet	Crosse & Blackwell	96	27
mustard	Epicure	23	6.5
sweet	Epicure	77	22
	Haywards	75	22
traditional	Crosse & Blackwell	25	7
Piccalilly	Safeway	14	4
Pickle see also brand names			
Pickle, sweet		*134*	*38*
Pickle, sweet	BHS	85	24
	Epicure	134	38
	Happy Farm	134	38
	Tesco	172	49
military	Haywards	130	37
Pickled dill cucumber	Tesco	14	4
Pickled gherkins	Crosse & Blackwell	2	
	Epicure	17	5
	Haywards	5	1.5
Pickled onions	BHS	14	4
	Epicure	14	4
	Haywards	16	4.5
	Safeway	23	6.5
	Tesco	18	5
silverskin	BHS	20	6
	Epicure	17	5
	Haywards	20	6
	Heinz	20	6

Product	Brand	Calories per 100g/ 100ml	Calories per oz/ pack/ portion
Pickled onions, **sweet**	Epicure	25	7
	Haywards	25	7
	Tesco	28	8
white	Crosse & Blackwell	2	
Pickled red cabbage	Epicure	12	3.5
	Haywards	10	3
	Tesco	14	4
Pickled walnuts	Epicure	69	20
	Haywards	80	23
Picnic	Cadbury's	499	141
Picnic eggs	St Michael	330	94
Picnic salad	BHS	129	37
Pies *see Chicken and ham, etc*			
Pigeon, roast		*230*	*65*
(with bone)		*101*	*29*
Pig liver *see Liver*			
Pilchard and tomato paste	Shippams	150	43
Pilchards in tomato sauce		*126*	*36*
Pilchards in tomato sauce	John West	138	39
Pineapple, canned		*77*	*22*
Pineapple, canned			
all shapes (drained)	Tesco	67	19
cubes or slices	Waitrose	77	22
rings in natural juice	John West	57	16
rings in syrup	Sainsbury		2 + 1 tbsp syrup 75

Product	Brand	Calories per 100g/ 100ml	Calories per oz/ pack/ portion
Pineapple, canned			
rings in syrup	John West	70	20
slices	BHS	70	20
	Libby	57	16
tidbits	Libby	58	16
Pineapple, fresh		*46*	*13*
Pineapple, fresh	Sainsbury	44	½in. slice/ 2oz 25
Pineapple cheesecake	St Michael	275	78
Pineapple crush	Slimsta	4.5	1.3
Pineapple dessert topping	Colman's	280	79
Pineapple flan filling	Armour	98	28
Pineapple jam	Hartley's	255	72
Pineapple jelly dessert (as sold)	Chivers	285	81
Pineapple juice (canned)		*53*	*15*
Pineapple juice	Britvic	52	15
	Heinz	57	16
	Libby	53	15
	Sainsbury	53	¼ pint 75
	St Michael	41	12
	Schweppes	48	14
	Tesco	42	12
	Waitrose	44	12
fresh	BHS	48	14
sweetened	Club	57	113ml 65
	Hunts	52	15
UHT	BHS	44	12

Product	Brand	Calories per 100g/ 100ml	Calories per oz/ pack/ portion
Pineapple Pavlova	Ross	270	77
Pineapple Rise and Shine	Kellogg's	333 (dry)	4fl.oz/114ml 50
Pineapple split	Wall's		each 90
Pineapple yogurt/ yoghurt	St Michael	83	24
	Ski	90	26
	Waitrose	95	27
Pint Size (as sold)	Cadbury's	480	136
Pistachios, dry roasted	Tesco	500	142
Pizza	Sainsbury	229	65
Pizza, bacon, mushroom and peppers	St Michael	182	52
Pizza, cheese and tomato		*234*	*66*
Pizza, cheese and tomato	St Michael	239	68
Pizza, French bread	BHS	238	130g 310
Pizza, ham and mushroom deep dish	St Michael	207	59
Pizza, Italian style sausage	St Michael	214	61
Pizza Marguerita (6 per pack)	St Michael	218	62
Pizza mix (as sold)	Whitworths	344	153g pack 520
Pizza Prima	BHS	265	265g 703
Pizza sauce (Prego), undiluted	Campbell's	76	22
Pizza Toast Topper	Heinz	70	20
Pizzalets	Peek Frean	493	per biscuit 11

Product	Brand	Calories per 100g/ 100ml	Calories per oz/ pack/ portion
PLAICE			
fresh fillets	St Michael	94	27
fresh whole boneless	St Michael	94	27
fresh or frozen	Sainsbury	70	20
fried in batter		279	79
fried in crumbs		228	65
frozen, fried	Waitrose	141	40
frozen, on the bone	Waitrose	49	14
frozen, smoked fillets	Waitrose	92	26
frozen fillet	Birds Eye	71	20
frozen fillets	BHS	80	23
	Ross	80	23
frozen fillets, breaded	BHS	130	37
frozen fillets, crispy (shallow fried)	Birds Eye	247	70
frozen fillets in breadcrumbs	Ross	140	40
frozen fillets in crisp crunch crumb (baked or grilled)	Birds Eye	229	65
frozen fillets in crisp crunch crumb (shallow fried)	Birds Eye	300	85
frozen whole crispy (fried)	Birds Eye	229	65
raw		91	26
rolled (2 per pack)	St Michael	117	33
steamed		93	26

Product	Brand	Calories per 100g/ 100ml	Calories per oz/ pack/ portion
PLAICE			
steamed (with bones and skin)		50	14
stuffed – mushroom and butter	St Michael	85	24
stuffed – mushroom and cheese	St Michael	120	34
stuffed – prawn and mushroom	St Michael	109	31
whole breaded, grilled or fried, brushed with a little oil first	Sainsbury	212	60
Plaice in breadcrumbs (2 small whole boneless, 2 fillets or 2lb bag)	St Michael	132	37
Plaice in cream sauce	Birds Eye		per pack 220
Plain chocolate see Chocolate			
Plain chocolate biscuit thins	St Michael	527	per biscuit 30
Plain chocolate coconut rings	Tesco	471	134
Plain chocolate crisps	St Michael	501	per biscuit 42
Plain chocolate digestive	Cadbury's	465	132
	Huntley & Palmers	490	per biscuit 61
	Sainsbury		per biscuit 70
half coat	St Michael	500	per biscuit 65

215

Product	Brand	Calories per 100g/ 100ml	Calories per oz/ pack/ portion
Plain chocolate fingers	Safeway	534	152
Plain chocolate flavour bar (cooking)	Tesco	308	87
Plain chocolate ginger biscuits	St Michael	490	per biscuit 64
Plain chocolate homewheat	McVitie		per biscuit 74
Plain chocolate mint wafers	BHS	510	145
Plain chocolate orange cream sandwich biscuits	Waitrose	518	147
Plain chocolate orange sandwich biscuits	Sainsbury		per biscuit 100
Plain chocolate orange wafers	BHS	510	145
Plain chocolate sweetmeal	BHS Tesco	500 499	142 141
Plain flour *see Flour*			
Plain Jane almond toffees, bag or loose	Callard & Bowser, Nuttall	480	per sweet 40
Plantain, green, boiled		*122*	*35*
raw		*112*	*32*
Plantain, ripe, fried		*267*	*76*
PLJ lemon cordial, low calorie (made up)	Beecham Foods	24	7

Product	Brand	Calories per 100g/100ml	Calories per pack/portion
PLJ lemon juice, original sharp (made up)	Beecham Foods	24	7
Ploughman's pasty	Kraft	306	142g/5oz pasty 435
Ploughman's pickle	Heinz	136	39
Plum jam	Safeway	263	75
	Tesco	279	79
	Waitrose	261	74
Plum pie filling	Pack-a-Pie	60	per pack 241
Plum yogurt	Ski	93	26
Plums, canned	Sainsbury		4+1 tbsp syrup 125
Plums, cooking			
raw		26	7.5
raw (with stones)		23	6.5
stewed with sugar		59	17
stewed with sugar (with stones)		55	16
stewed without sugar		22	6
stewed without sugar (with stones)		20	6
Plums, fresh	Sainsbury	35	1×2oz 20
Plums, Victoria dessert,		38	11
raw (with stones)		36	10
Poacher's Broth	Baxters	42	15oz/425g can 177
Polo, milk chocolate	Tesco	496	141

Product	Brand	Calories per 100g/ 100ml	Calories per oz/ pack/ portion
Polo Fruits	Rowntree Mackintosh	380	per pack 105
Polo Peppermints	Rowntree Mackintosh	400	per pack 100
Polony		*281*	*80*
Pomagne, dry	H.P. Bulmer	53	15
sweet	H.P. Bulmer	66	19
Pomegranate juice		*44*	*12*
Pommia, dry	Taunton	53	1 pint 53
sweet	Taunton	65	1 pint 380
Pontefract cakes	Bassett's	286	81
Popcorn	St Michael	334	95
	Tesco	390	111
PORK			
belly rashers, grilled, lean and fat		*398*	*113*
raw, lean and fat		*381*	*108*
boneless shoulder	St Michael	251	71
chops	St Michael	329	93
grilled, lean and fat	Sainsbury	165	1 chop/6oz 280
grilled, lean only	Sainsbury	85	1 chop/6oz 145
dressed carcase, raw		*338*	*96*
escalopes	St Michael	147	42
fat, cooked (average)		*619*	*175*
raw, (average)		*670*	*190*
kebabs	St Michael	175	50

Product	Brand	Calories per 100g/ 100ml	Calories per oz/ pack/ portion
PORK			
lean, raw (average)		*147*	*42*
leg, raw, lean and fat		*269*	*76*
roast, lean and fat		*286*	*81*
roast, lean and fat	Sainsbury	282	1 slice/2oz 160
roast, lean only		*185*	*52*
roast, lean only	Sainsbury	194	1 slice/2oz 110
loin chops, grilled, lean and fat		*332*	*94*
grilled, lean and fat (with bone)		*258*	*73*
grilled, lean only		*226*	*64*
grilled, lean only (with bone)		*133*	*38*
raw		*329*	*93*
loin joint, Danish smoked cured	St Michael	140	40
steaks in breadcrumbs	St Michael	279	79
Pork, canned			
cured	St Michael	270	77
shoulder	Sainsbury	123	1 slice/1oz 35
Pork, sliced meats			
pressed tongue	St Michael	171	48
shoulder	St Michael	125	35
smoked loin	St Michael	200	57
Pork and apple pasty	BHS	467	155g pasty 725

219

Product	Brand	Calories per 100g/ 100ml	Calories per oz/ pack/ portion
Pork and beef chipolatas	Tesco	328	93
Pork and beef sausages	Ross	280	79
	Sainsbury	317	1, 2oz raw 180, grilled 130
(8 per pack)	BHS	366	per lb 1660
jumbo	Ross	280	79
	Tesco	313	89
medium or large (8 or 12 per lb)	Tesco	315	89
skinless	St Michael	338	96
	Tesco	342	97
standard	St Michael	333	94
Pork and egg pie, sliced	St Michael	385	109
Pork and herb sausages (8 per pack)	BHS	352	per lb 1600
	Tesco	376	107
Pork and liver pâté	BHS	324	92
Pork and mushroom pâté	BHS	322	91
Pork and tomato sausages (8 per pack)	BHS	386	per lb 1750
Pork breakfast sausage	Sainsbury	247	3 slices/1oz 70
Pork chipolatas	Tesco	358	101
	Waitrose	342	97

Product	Brand	Calories per 100g/ 100ml	Calories per oz/ pack/ portion
Pork cocktail sausages	Tesco	393	111
Pork kidneys, braised (canned)	Tesco	100	28
Pork liver pâté	Princes	316	90
Pork loin (cooked)	BHS	120	34
Pork luncheon meat (canned)	Waitrose	335	95
	Sainsbury	265	1 slice/1oz 75
	Tesco	321	91
(sliced)	Sainsbury	282	80
Pork pâté	Country Pot	155	44
Pork pie (individual)		*376*	*107*
Pork pie (¼oz)	Sainsbury	368	per pie 470
(10oz)	Sainsbury	349	per pie 990
(16oz)	Sainsbury	352	¼ pie/4oz 400
(1½lb)	BHS	456	per pie 3100
(pack of 4)	St Michael	435	123
buffet	Tesco	459	130
country style	Tesco	486	138
crisp bake, large (16oz)	St Michael	377	107
crisp bake, large flat	St Michael	337	96
crisp bake, small (2 or 4 per pack)	St Michael	382	108
crusty bake	Sainsbury	388	3½oz pie 385
farmhouse	BHS	372	10oz pie 1056
farmhouse flat	BHS	356	1lb pie 1616
Lincolnshire	BHS	448	7oz pie 890
		463	1lb pie 2100

221

Product	Brand	Calories per 100g/ 100ml	Calories per oz/ pack/ portion
Pork pie			
mini	Sainsbury	388	2oz pie 220
party	BHS	406	68g pie 276
picnic	BHS	321	12oz pie 1092
savoury	Safeway	350	100
traditional	Tesco	328	93
Pork piquant Casserole Mix (as sold)	Colman's	295	84
Pork sausages	Ross	300	85
	Safeway	355	101
	Sainsbury	370	1, 2oz raw 210 grilled 150
	Waitrose	342	97
(8 per pack)	BHS	326	92
	Tesco	342	97
flavoured with sage and onion	St Michael	433	123
premium	Tesco	308	87
skinless	Birds Eye		each, fried or grilled 70
	Sainsbury	353	1, 1oz raw 100 grilled 70
	Tesco	342	97
	Waitrose	342	97
smoked (8 per pack)	Tesco	358	101
standard	St Michael	437	124
top quality	BHS	350	99
	St Michael	440	125
in lard (canned)	Tesco	312	88

Product	Brand	Calories per 100g/100ml	Calories per oz/pack/portion
Pork shoulder	BHS	125	141g pack 177
Porkburgers (fresh)	Tesco	280	79
Porridge		*44*	*12*
Porridge, instant (as sold)	Waitrose	405	115
Porridge made with 2 tbsp oatmeal and 8 tbsp water	Sainsbury	77	1 tbsp/½oz 11
Porridge, wheatmeal	Prewetts	335	95
Porridge oats	BHS	355	101
	Tesco	402	114
	Waitrose	405	115
	Whitworths	401	114 raw
		44	12 cooked
Port		*157*	*45*
Port Salut cheese	Tesco	313	89
Pot Noodles, Pot Rice see under flavours			
Potato and leek soup (undiluted)	Granny's	43	12
Potato and smoked bacon salad	BHS	291	82
Potato Bake, sliced potato	St Michael	107	30
Potato cakes	St Michael	183	52
Potato chips (snack)	Sainsbury	500	125
Potato crisps see also under flavours			
Potato crisps		*533*	*151*
Potato crisps	Sainsbury	500	25g 125
Potato croquettes	Birds Eye		each, baked 30, fried 50

223

Product	Brand	Calories per 100g/ 100ml	Calories per oz/ pack/ portion
Potato croquettes	BHS	118	454g pack 538
	Ross	110	30
	Sainsbury		each 20
Potato fritters, crispy (fried or grilled)	Birds Eye	194	55
Potato noisettes (as sold)	Ross	170	50
Potato rings	St Michael	516	146
	Tesco	533	151
Potato salad	Eden Vale	146	41
	St Michael	322	91
	Tesco	145	41
(canned)	Heinz	191	54
	Sainsbury	141	1 tbsp/1oz 40
	Tesco	155	44
with chives	Sainsbury	176	1 tbsp/1oz 50
Potato scallops	BHS	182	2lb pack 1658
Potato sticks	BHS	505	143
	St Michael	505	143
	Waitrose	550	156
Potato swirls	Sainsbury	420	105
Potato thins	St Michael	501	142
Potato twirls	Safeway	423	121
Potato waffles	Birds Eye		each, baked or grilled 80, fried 120
POTATOES			
baked		105	30
(with skins)		85	24
boiled		80	23

224

Product	Brand	Calories per 100g/ 100ml	Calories per oz/ pack/ portion
POTATOES			
canned	Napolina	64	18
	Yeoman	68	19
chipped see Chips			
instant powder		*318*	*90*
made up		*70*	*20*
Jersey (canned)	Tesco	78	22
	Waitrose	74	21
mashed		*119*	*34*
new (boiled)		*76*	*22*
(canned)		*53*	*15*
raw		*87*	*25*
roast		*157*	*45*
Pour Over Sauces see under flavours			
Praline éclairs	St Michael	470	133
Prawn cocktail crisps	St Michael	536	152
	Tesco	560	159
Prawn cocktail sauce	Colman's	390	111
	Safeway	390	111
	Tesco	320	91
Prawn cocktail snacks	St Michael	486	138
	Tesco	487	138
Prawn curry	Birds Eye		per pack 180
	Vesta	331	per pack 642
Prawn curry Knoodles	Knorr	355	101
Prawn Provençale Knoodles	Knorr	366	104
Prawn salad	Eden Vale	153	43
	St Ivel	155	44
	Tesco	101	29

Product	Brand	Calories per 100g/ 100ml	Calories per oz/ pack/ portion
Prawn shells	BHS	486	138
Prawns			
boiled		107	30
(with shells)		41	12
canned	Armour	94	27
	John West	86	24
frozen	BHS	106	113g pack 120
			226g pack 240
peeled	St Michael	107	30
Prego sauces see under flavours			
Princess biscuits	Macfarlane Lang		per biscuit 50
Priory biscuits	Huntley & Palmers	459	per biscuit 45
Private Label salad cream	HP Foods	320	91
Prize	Rowntree Mackintosh	450	per pack 225
Prize yogurt, fruit (average)	St Ivel	79	22
hazelnut	St Ivel	87	25
Processed cheese	Sainsbury	370	105
Family Favourites (average)	St Ivel	280	79
full fat	Waitrose	374	106
Gold Spinner	St Ivel	280	79
Swiss Knight assorted variety pack	Nestlé	321	91
Swiss Knight assorted variety pack cheese spreads	Nestlé	283	80

Product	Brand	Calories per 100g/ 100ml	Calories per oz/ pack/ portion
Processed cheese			
Swiss Knight			
medium fat	Nestlé	321	91
Swiss Knight slices/			
cheese spread	Nestlé	306	87
Processed peas *see Peas*			
Profiteroles (frozen)	BHS	312	88
Protose	Granose	159	45
Provençale			
Cooking-In sauce	Baxters	94	425g can 398
Provençale Master			
Sauce (as sold)	Colman's	325	92
Prune yoghurt	St Michael	101	29
Prunes			
canned (drained)	Tesco	109	31
canned (inc. syrup)	Hartley's	125	35
dried			
raw		*161*	*46*
raw (with stones)		*134*	*38*
stewed with sugar		*104*	*29*
stewed with sugar			
(with stones)		*95*	*27*
stewed without sugar		*82*	*23*
stewed without sugar			
(with stones)		*74*	*21*
dried	Sainsbury	141	4/1oz 40
	Tesco	122	35
	Whitworths	134	38
dried (with stones)	Safeway	134	38
dried, ready			
cooked	Whitworths	114	32

Product	Brand	Calories per 100g/ 100ml	Calories per oz/ pack/ portion
Puffa Puffa Rice	Kellogg's	410	116
Puffed rice	Tesco	375	106
Puffed wheat		*325*	*92*
Puffed Wheat	Quaker Oats	337	96
	Sainsbury	353	4 tbsp/½oz 50
Puffin, milk chocolate	Tesco	325	92
Pumpkin, raw		*15*	*4.5*

Product	Brand	Calories per 100g/ 100ml	Calories per oz/ pack/ portion
Quaker Oats	Quaker Oats	403	114
Queen of puddings		216	61
Queen Victoria sponge (frozen)	Lyons	328	per cake 909
Quench:	Lyons Maid		
cider			each 34
cola			each 38
Quiche Lorraine		391	111
Quick fry	Sainsbury	265	75
Quick oats	Tesco	413	117
Quick whip	Sainsbury		pkt made up 680
Quinces, raw		25	7
Quosh drinks *see under flavours*			

Product	Brand	Calories per 100g/ 100ml	Calories per oz/ pack/ portion
Rabbit			
raw		*124*	*35*
stewed		*179*	*51*
stewed (with bone)		*91*	*26*
Radishes, raw		*15*	*4.5*
Rainbow crystal sugar	Tesco	394	112
Rainbow trout			
(2 per pack)	St Michael	88	25
(2 per pack, frozen)	BHS	86	per pack 200
pink	St Michael	88	25
Raisin and bran tea loaf	St Michael	247	70
Raisin and brazil nut yoghurt	Waitrose	95	27
Raisin cake, spiced	St Michael	348	99
Raisins, dried		*246*	*70*
Raisins, dried	Safeway	247	70
	Sainsbury	247	1 tbsp/1oz 70
	Waitrose	247	70
seedless	Tesco	246	70
	Whitworths	246	70
stoned	Whitworths	246	70
Raspberries, canned		*87*	*25*
Raspberries			
canned	Baxters	86	10½oz/290g can 249
			15oz/425g can 366
			19oz/538g can 464
canned (inc. syrup)	Hartley's	85	24

230

Product	Brand	Calories per 100g/ 100ml	Calories per oz/ pack/ portion
Raspberries			
canned (inc. syrup)	Sainsbury	88	1 tbsp/1oz 25
fresh, raw		25	7
stewed with sugar		68	19
stewed without sugar		26	7.5
fresh or frozen	Sainsbury	22	1 tbsp/1oz 6
frozen	Waitrose	25	7
Raspberry and redcurrant pies	St Michael	341	per pie 182
Raspberry and redcurrant tarts	Sainsbury		per tart 270
Raspberry blancmange mix (as sold)	Brown & Polson	328	33g pack 108
Raspberry conserve	BHS	260	74
Raspberry creams	Pennywise		per biscuit 47
Raspberry Delight (made up)	Tesco	134	38
Raspberry dessert sauce	HP Foods	110	31
	Lyons Maid	266	75
	Tesco	323	92
	Wall's	110	250g pack 275
Raspberry dessert topping	Colman's	280	79
Raspberry drink	Zing	44	12
Raspberry flan filling	Armour	119	34
Raspberry jam	Chivers		
	Extra	250	71
	Hartley's	265	75
	Moorhouse	260	74

231

Product	Brand	Calories per 100g/ 100ml	Calories per oz/ pack/ portion
Raspberry jam	Robertson's	251	71
	Safeway	255	73
	Tesco	279	79
	Tesco Extra	268	76
	Waitrose	261	74
seedless	Hartley's	265	75
	Moorhouse	265	75
Raspberry jelly	Chivers	260	74
dessert (as sold)	Waitrose	258	73
Raspberry Jelly Cream	Chivers	370	105
Raspberry meringue	St Michael	297	84
Raspberry pie (4 portion)	Sainsbury		$\frac{1}{4}$ pie 250
Raspberry pie filling	Sainsbury	106	1tbsp/2oz 60
Raspberry preserve	Baxters	253	12oz/340g jar 860
Today's Recipe	Robertson's	180	51
Raspberry ripple	Tudor	170	48
	Wall's	175	180g pack 315 277g pack 480
family brick	Lyons Maid		per pack 432
handy pack	Lyons Maid		per pack 297
Soft Scoop (2 litre)	Wall's		per pack 2085
Soft Serve	Tudor	180	51
sliceable (588g/1 litre)	Wall's	173	per pack 1020
Raspberry ripple mousse	Tesco	162	46
Raspberry Romana Italiano (543g/1 litre)	Wall's	168	per pack 915

Product	Brand	Calories per 100g/ 100ml	Calories per oz/ pack/ portion
Raspberry Royale	St Michael	133	38
Raspberry sponge pudding	Heinz	282	80
Raspberry sponge sandwich	Lyons	326	per cake 750
Raspberry supermousse	Birds Eye		per tub 120
Raspberry Two Shakes	Kellogg's	359 (dry)	½ sachet (20g) + ½ pint milk 273
Raspberry yogurt/ yoghurt	St Michael	101	29
	Ski	92	26
	Waitrose	95	27
Raspberry/redcurrant pies	Waitrose	198	56
Ratatouille	Buitoni	39	11
	St Michael	85	24
	Tesco	33	9.5
Ravioli	Buitoni	73	21
	Granose	64	18
	Sainsbury	106	1tbsp/1oz 30
in beef and tomato sauce	Heinz	90	26
in tomato sauce	Heinz	96	27
	Tesco	70	20
Ready Brek		*390*	*111*
Ready dinner	Goblin	100	425g pack 425
Ready salted crisps	BHS	550	25g pack 137
	St Michael	545	155
	Tesco	545	155
	Waitrose	550	156

233

Product	Brand	Calories per 100g/ 100ml	Calories per oz/ pack/ portion
Ready salted sticks	Tesco	505	143
Ready to bake white rolls	St Michael	271	77
Real fruit centres	BHS	354	150g pack 531
Real fruit jellies (carton)	Clarnico		per pack 660 per sweet 30
Real milk ice	Lyons Maid		each 50
Red cabbage, pickled	Epicure	12	3.5
	Haywards	10	3
	Tesco	14	4
Red cherry yoghurt	Waitrose	95	27
Red kidney beans	Batchelors	74	21
	Whitworths	272	77
Red Leicester cheese	Prewetts	391	111
	Tesco	388	110
Red plum jam	Hartley's	260	74
	Moorhouse	255	72
Red Stripe strong lager	H.P. Bulmer	45	13
Red wine see **Wine**			
Red wine Cook-in-Sauce	Homepride	77	376g pack 290
Red wine Pour Over sauce	Crosse & Blackwell	37	10
Redcurrant and raspberry pie filling	Pack-a-Pie	74	per pack 299
Redcurrant jelly	Hartley's	265	75
	Crosse & Blackwell	259	73
Redcurrant sauce	Colman's	290	82

234

Product	Brand	Calories per 100g/ 100ml	Calories per oz/ pack/ portion
Redcurrants			
raw		21	6
stewed with sugar		53	15
stewed without sugar		18	5
Refreshers	Trebor		per pack 100 per sweet 6.5
Revels	Mars		standard pack 183 per sweet 8–16
Rhubarb			
raw		6	2
stewed with sugar		45	13
stewed without sugar		6	2
Rhubarb			
canned	Safeway	70–80	20–23
canned drained	Tesco	60	17
canned (inc. syrup)	Hartley's	60	17
	Sainsbury	75	1tbsp/1oz 21
fresh	Sainsbury	4	1
Rhubarb and ginger preserve	Baxters	260	12oz/340g jar 884
Rhubarb tart (large)	St Michael	185	52
Ribena (undiluted)		229	65
Ribena	Beecham Foods	292	83
Baby		318	90
Rice *see also Savoury, etc*			
Rice			
polished, boiled		123	35
polished, raw		361	102

Product	Brand	Calories per 100g/ 100ml	Calories per oz/ pack/ portion
RICE (raw)	Sainsbury	353	1tbsp/1oz 100
(all types)	Safeway	361	102
basmati	Whitworths	363	103
boil in the bag	Kellogg's	327	93
brown	Whitworths	360	102
easy cook	Tesco	353	100
	Waitrose	360	102
	Whitworths	369	105
ground	Whitworths	363	103
long grain	Tesco	356	101
	Waitrose	360	102
	Whitworths	363	103
natural	Uncle Ben's	355	101
short or round grain (pudding)	Tesco	356	101
	Waitrose	360	102
	Whitworths	363	103
unpolished (long or short grain)	Prewetts	340	96
white	Uncle Ben's	350	100
Rice, peas and mushrooms	Birds Eye	123 boiled	35 boiled
Rice, sweetcorn and peppers	Birds Eye	123 boiled	35 boiled
Rice & Things see under flavours			
Rice Creamola	Rowntree Mackintosh	355	101
Rice crisp	Sainsbury	476	1/5 cake /1oz 135

Product	Brand	Calories per 100g/ 100ml	Calories per oz/ pack/ portion
Rice crisp	St Michael	321	per cake 92
	Waitrose	554	157
Rice crisps	BHS	464	140g pack 650
Rice dessert (2 per pack)	St Michael	179	51
Rice Krispies		*372*	*105*
Rice Krispies	Kellogg's	345	98
Rice pudding, canned		*91*	*26*
Rice pudding			
canned	Sainsbury	112	15½oz can 490
	Tesco	87	25
creamed, canned	Ambrosia	94	27
	Libby	89	25
	Safeway	144	45
	Waitrose	148	42
creamed ground rice	Ambrosia	90	26
traditional	Ambrosia	107	30
Rich Danish shortcake	BHS	520	147
Rich fruit cake,			
all butter	St Michael	353	100
iced top	St Michael	310	88
Rich fruit pudding (canned)	Sainsbury	336	10½oz can 1000
Rich Highland Shorties	Meredith & Drew		per biscuit 50
Rich shortie biscuits	Tesco	500	142
Rich tea biscuits	McVitie		per biscuit 33
	Peek Frean	436	per biscuit 25
	Sainsbury		per biscuit 50

Product	Brand	Calories per 100g/ 100ml	Calories per oz/ pack/ portion
Rich tea biscuits	Waitrose	582	165
(all shapes)	Tesco	466	132
round	BHS	459	130
	St Michael	460	per biscuit 45
Rich tea finger creams	St Michael	484	per biscuit 51
chocolate flavour	St Michael	498	per biscuit 52
Rich tea fingers	St Michael	459	per biscuit 23
Ricicles	Kellogg's	351	100
Ring biscuits, iced		448	127
Ring mallows	Peek Frean	384	per biscuit 49
Ripple, single	Mars		per pack 141
Rise and Shine *see under flavours*			
Rissole mix	Prewetts	408	172
Rissoles, savoury	Birds Eye		each, fried or grilled 190
Rissolnut	Granose	376	107
Roast beef dinner	Birds Eye		per pack 360
Roasted almond bar, Bourneville	Cadbury's	534	151
Rock around the Choc	Lyons Maid		each 129
Rock cakes		394	112
Rocket (multipack)	Lyons Maid		each 29
Roe, cod (hard), raw		113	32
fried		202	57
Roe, herring (soft), raw		80	23
fried		244	69
Rogan Josh Classic Curry	Homepride	104	383g pack 400
Rolls *see Bread rolls*			

Product	Brand	Calories Per 100g/ 100ml	Calories per oz/ pack/ portion
Rolo	Rowntree	450	per pack 230
Rosé wine see **Wine**			
Rosehip syrup, undiluted		*232*	*66*
Roses Assortment	Cadbury's	443	126
Rose's Juices see **Lemon, etc**			
Round bun	Sainsbury		¼ bun 145
Royal Game soup	Baxters	32	per can 138
Royal Scot biscuits	McVitie		per biscuit 54
Royale desserts see **under flavours**			
Rum and raisin fudge	Callard & Bowser	410	per bar 225
Rum Babas	St Michael	234	per cake 210
Rum liqueur bar	St Michael	467	132
Rump steak see **Beef**			
Runner beans, sliced (canned)	Waitrose	18	5
Russchian	Schweppes	22	6
Ry King crispbread:	McVitie		
brown			per piece 33
light			per piece 28
wheat			per piece 38
Rye crispbread	Primula	312	per piece 22
	Sainsbury		per piece 30
extra thin	Sainsbury		per piece 20
whole rye	Tesco	375	106
Rye flour	Prewetts	339	96
Rye-bran crispbread:	Primula		
extra thin		261	per piece 12
thick		261	per piece 21

Product	Brand	Calories per 100g/ 100ml	Calories per oz/ pack/ portion
Safflower seed oil	Alfonal	900	255
Sage, rubbed	Tesco	350	99
Sage and onion Coat & Cook	Homepride	453	43g pack 195
Sage and onion stuffing	Tesco	346	98
	Whitworths	382	108
Sage Derby cheese	Sainsbury	370	105
Sago (raw)		355	*101*
Sago (raw)	Safeway	355	101
	Whitworths	355	101
Sago pudding	Whitworths	131	37
canned	Sainsbury	91	15½oz can 400
creamed, canned	Ambrosia	88	25
St Paulin cheese	Sainsbury	300	85
Saithe			
raw		73	*21*
steamed		99	*28*
steamed (with bones and skin)		84	*24*
Salad cream		311	*88*
Salad cream	BHS	315	89
	Crosse & Blackwell	392	111
	Heinz	312	88
	HP Foods	320	91
	Safeway	392	111
	Sainsbury	194	1 tbsp/1oz 55
	Tesco	402	114
Salad Days *see under flavours*			
Salad dressing	Alfonal	310	88

Product	Brand	Calories per 100g/ 100ml	Calories per oz/ pack/ portion
Salads *see Coleslaw, etc*			
Salami		*491*	*139*
Salami	BHS	430	122
	St Michael	491	139
country-style	BHS	430	122
Danish	Sainsbury	546	155
Salmon, canned		*155*	*44*
Salmon, canned	Armour	155	44
	Sainsbury	123	35
medium red	John West	167	47
pink	John West	140	40
red	Waitrose	137	39
	John West	210	60
Salmon, fresh			
raw		*182*	*52*
steamed		*197*	*56*
steamed (with bones and skin)		*160*	*45*
Salmon, sliced Scotch	BHS	180	51
Salmon, smoked		*142*	*40*
Salmon, smoked	St Michael	142	40
Salmon and cucumber paste	Princes	114	32
Salmon and shrimp paste (35g g or 78g)	Shippams	170	48
Salmon and shrimp spread	Princes	104	29
Salmon pâté	John West	210	60
	Shippams	175	50
with mayonnaise	Country Pot	190	54
Salmon spread	Princes	121	34

Product	Brand	Calories per 100g/ 100ml	Calories per oz/ pack/ portion
Salsify, boiled		*18*	*5*
Salt, block or table		*nil*	
Salt and vinegar chiplets	St Michael	487	138
Salt and vinegar chips	BHS	505	143
Salt and vinegar crisps	BHS	530	150
	Safeway	559	158
	Sainsbury	520	25g 130
	St Michael	523	148
	Tesco	527	149
	Waitrose	550	156
Salt and vinegar moons	Tesco	480	136
Salt and vinegar sticks	Tesco	473	134
Salted cashews	Sainsbury	564	160
	Sun-Pat	585	166
Salted crisps	Safeway	559	158
Salted mixed nuts	Sun-Pat	605	172
Salted peanuts	BHS	570	162
	Sainsbury	600	170
	Sun-Pat	600	170
Samsoe cheese (45% fat in the dry matter)	Danish	344	98
Sandwich biscuits		*513*	*145*
Sandwich biscuit	Cadbury's	510	144
Sandwich creams	Sainsbury		per biscuit 65
Sandwich Spread	Heinz	240	68

Product	Brand	Calories per 100g/ 100ml	Calories per oz/ pack/ portion
Sardine and tomato paste (78g)	Shippams	160	45
Sardine and tomato spread (35g)	Shippams	170	48
Sardine spread with tomato	Country Pot	160	45
Sardines in oil			
fish only		217	62
fish plus oil		334	95
Sardines in oil (fish only)	Armour	217	62
	John West	197	56
	Tesco	295	84
Sardines in tomato sauce		177	50
Sardines in tomato sauce	Armour	177	50
	John West	177	50
	Tesco	220	62
Sauce Provençale (Cooking-In)	Baxters	94	425g can 398
Sauce Tartare see Tartare			
Sausage meat	BHS	374	per lb 1700
beef and pork	Sainsbury	353	100
pork	Tesco	345	98
pork and beef	Tesco	313	89
pork and herbs	Tesco	371	105
Sausage rolls			
flaky pastry		479	136
short pastry		463	131

Product	Brand	Calories per 100g/ 100ml	Calories per oz/ pack/ portion
Sausage rolls	Birds Eye		per roll, 150 baked 145
	Ross	310	88
	Tiffany's	265	per roll 130
(160g pack)	BHS	812	per pack 1300
(pack of 6)	BHS		per pack 663
cheese pastry (28g/1oz)	Kraft Cheese Fayre	268	per roll 75
cocktail (28g/1oz)	Kraft	392	per roll 110
jumbo	Ross	310	88
king size (57g/2oz)	Kraft	377	per roll 215
large	Sainsbury	414	1×2oz 235
lattice, with onion	BHS	348	206g pack 718
mini	Sainsbury	440	1×0.8oz 100
plain	Tesco	412	117
puff pastry, pork	St Michael	390	111
puff pastry, pork and beef	St Michael	519	147
savoury	Sainsbury	428	1×0.7oz 85
Sausages, for brands see under Beef, Pork, etc			
Sausages, beef			
fried		269	76
grilled		265	75
raw		299	85
Sausages, Continental see Bierwurst, etc			
Sausages, pork			
fried		317	90
grilled		318	90
raw		367	104
Sausalatas	Granose	137	39

Product	Brand	Calories per 100g/ 100ml	Calories per oz/ pack/ portion
Sausalene	Granose	195	55
Sausfry	Granose	492	139
Saveloy		262	74
Saviand	Granose	199	56
Savoree sausage	Sainsbury	265	75
Savours (round)	McVitie		per biscuit 22
Savoury beef and onion soup	Batchelors 5-Minute		per pack 154
Savoury beef Pot Rice	Golden Wonder		carton made up 254
Savoury crackers	Waitrose	596	169
Savoury curried rice (made up)	Crosse & Blackwell	105	30
Savoury faggots	Sainsbury	282	80
Savoury minced beef with onions in gravy	Fray Bentos	120	34
Savoury mix, 5-cereal	Prewetts	341	97
Savoury pork pie	Safeway	350	100
Savoury pudding	Granose	207	59
Savoury puffs	Safeway	595	169
	St Michael	600	170
	Waitrose	529	150
Savoury rice (as sold):	Batchelors		
beef flavour		310	per pack 406
chicken flavour		340	per pack 435
golden		342	per pack 438
mild curry		332	per pack 451
mixed vegetable		343	per pack 446
sweet and sour		348	per pack 501

Product	Brand	Calories per 100g/ 100ml	Calories per oz/ pack/ portion
Savoury rice (as sold):	Tesco		
beef		345	98
chicken		350	99
hot curry		334	95
mild curry		327	93
mixed vegetable		334	95
saffron/golden		332	94
tomato		329	93
Savoury rice and mushrooms (made up)	Crosse & Blackwell Rice & Things	106	30
Savoury rice and peppers (made up)	Crosse & Blackwell Rice & Things	106	30
Savoury rice and vegetables (made up)	Crosse & Blackwell Rice & Things	105	30
Savoury rissoles (as sold)	Tiffany's	250	per rissole 125
Savoury spread yeast extract	Safeway	190	55
Savoury vegetable soup	Batchelors 5-Minute		per pack 19
Savoy biscuits	Huntley & Palmers	505	per biscuit
Scallops, jacket (as sold)	Ross	120	35
steamed		105	30

Product	Brand	Calories per 100g/ 100ml	Calories per oz/ pack/ portion
Scampi			
fried		*316*	*90*
golden, frozen	BHS	165	284g pack 470 (sauce 150)
in breadcrumbs	Sainsbury	317	90
in breadcrumbs, large bag (no sauce)	St Michael	151	43
Scampi soup *see Cream of scampi*			
Scones		*371*	*105*
Scones	Sainsbury		per scone 130
fresh cream	St Michael	340	per scone 180
Scotch beef broth	Baxters	41	15oz/425g can 171
Scotch broth			
canned	Baxters	42	15oz/425g can 180
	BHS	40	11
	Crosse & Blackwell	62	18
	Heinz Big Soups	66	19
	Heinz Ready to Serve	40	11
	Waitrose	37	11
condensed (undiluted)	Campbell's Bumper Harvest	44	12
	Campbell's Condensed	61	17

247

Product	Brand	Calories per 100g/ 100ml	Calories per oz/ pack/ portion
Scotch broth	Granny's	52	15
dried (as sold)	5-Minute		per pack 137
	Tesco	345	98
dried (made up)	Sainsbury	21	½ pint 60
low calorie	Heinz	21	6
Scotch butter shortbread	Waitrose	522	148
Scotch crumpets	St Michael	298	84
Scotch eggs		279	79
Scotch eggs	Safeway	264	76
	Sainsbury	172	1×4oz 195
	St Michael	300	85
Scotch fritters with beans	Ross	240	68
with cheese	Ross	250	71
Scotch ginger cake	Sainsbury	300	¹/₇ cake/2oz 170
Scotch herring in tomato sauce	Crosse & Blackwell	154	44
Scotch mince	Baxters	110	15½oz/432g can 476
Scotch orange marmalade	Baxters	260	12oz/340g jar 884
Scotch pancakes		283	80
Scotch pancakes	Sainsbury		each 70
	St Michael	304	86
Scotch pies	St Michael	251	71
Scotch vegetable soup	Baxters	26	15oz/425g can 112
	BHS	26	7.5

248

Product	Brand	Calories per 100g/ 100ml	Calories per oz/ pack/ portion
Scottish haggis	Baxters	170	14½oz/411g can 699
Scottish lentil soup with vegetable	Crosse & Blackwell	45	13
Scottish vegetable soup with lentils	Heinz	59	17
Screwball – 2 Ball	Wall's		each 115
Sea Food Pasta	St Michael	121	34
Seafood and chicken paella	Birds Eye		pack cooked with knob of butter 340
Seafood platter (frozen)	BHS	200	per pack 453
Seafood sauce	Waistline	134	38
Seakale, boiled		8	2.5
Select orange marmalade	Rose's	260	74
Self-raising flour see *Flour*			
Semolina (raw)		350	99
Semolina (raw)	James Marshall	320	91
	Waitrose	353	100
	Whitworths	350	99
Semolina pudding canned	Whitworths	131	37
	Sainsbury	91	15½oz can 400
creamed, canned	Ambrosia	90	26
Sesame and sunflower biscuits	Prewetts	535	152
Seven-Up	Schweppes	38	11

Product	Brand	Calories per 100g/ 100ml	Calories per oz/ pack/ portion
Seville orange marmalade	Waitrose	258	74
Shandy	Barr	26	7.5
	BHS	29	8
	Club	22	185ml 40
	Corona	25	7
	Idris	25	7
	Slimsta	6	2
Shepherd's pie		*119*	*34*
Shepherd's pie cheesey topped (454g/16oz)	Sainsbury Kraft Cheese	174	16oz pie 790
	Fayre	154	per pie 700
family	Brains		per pie 555
	Ross	100	28
frozen	Birds Eye	119	8oz pie 270
	Ross	120	34
	Tesco	110	31
Sherbet fruits	BHS	396	150g pack 594
Sherbet lemons	Trebor		per sweet 25
Sherbet monsters	Lyons Maid		each 48
Sherbet powder	Bassett's	367	104
Sherry			
dry		*116*	*33*
medium		*118*	*33*
sweet		*136*	*39*
Sherry, dry	Sainsbury		sm. glass/ 1/3 gill 50
medium			sm. glass/ 1/3 gill 55
sweet			sm. glass/ 1/3 gill 60

Product	Brand	Calories per 100g/ 100ml	Calories per oz/ pack/ portion
Shoulder (cold meat)	Waitrose	423	120
Shortbread		*504*	*143*
Shortbread	Paterson's	500	142
Scotch butter	Waitrose	522	148
wholemeal	Allinson	494	140
Shortbread fingers	Sainsbury		per finger 90
	St Michael	517	per finger 109
	Waitrose	522	148
all butter	BHS	496	141
Shortbread Highland fingers	Crawford		per finger 64
Shortcake biscuits	McVitie		per biscuit 63
	Peek Frean	488	per biscuit 51
	Sainsbury		per biscuit 45
	Waitrose	504	143
milk chocolate	Tesco	513	145
petticoat	Tesco	510	145
plain	Tesco	501	142
thick	Sainsbury		per biscuit 65
Shortcake snack	Cadbury's	514	146
Shorties	Cadbury's	495	140
	Peek Frean	480	per biscuit 44
	Pennywise		per biscuit 38
	Sainsbury		per biscuit 45
	St Michael	494	per biscuit 55
Shredded Wheat		*324*	*92*
Shrimps, boiled		*117*	*33*
(with shells)		*39*	*11*
canned		*94*	*27*
Shrimps, canned	Armour	94	27
	John West	91	26

Product	Brand	Calories per 100g/ 100ml	Calories per oz/ pack/ portion
Sild			
in oil (drained)	John West	227	64
	Tesco	273	77
in tomato sauce	John West	172	49
	Tesco	203	58
Silky Smooth choc ice	Lyons Maid		each 132
Silver Shred	Robertson's	251	71
Silverside *see Beef*			
Silverskin onions *see Pickled onions*			
Singles (cheese slices)	Kraft	310	88
Sirloin *see Beef*			
Sizzles	St Michael	455	129
Skate, fried in batter		*199*	*56*
fried (with waste)		*163*	*46*
Skim milk, made up	Sainsbury	35	1 tbsp 5, ¼ pint 50
Skim milk powder	Sainsbury		1 tbsp 25
Ski yogurt:	Eden Vale		
banana		96	27
black cherry		94	27
hazelnut		100	28
orange		93	26
peach		96	27
peach melba		91	26
pear		95	27
pineapple		90	26
plum		93	26
raspberry		92	26
strawberry		91	26
Skull	Lyons Maid		each 80

Product	Brand	Calories per 100g/ 100ml	Calories per oz/ pack/ portion
Slender (as sold)	Carnation	361	102
Slender Slim			
chocolate	Carnation	365	11g svg 40
chocolate or	Carnation	360	22.5g svg
strawberry sweet			80
Slender Slim soups	Carnation	334	12g svg 40
Slender Slim Start:	Carnation		
grapefruit		345	14.5g svg 50
orange		323	15.5g svg 50
Slim-a-Soup *see flavours*			
Slimway low calorie			
dressing	Heinz	130	37
mayonnaise	Heinz	353	100
Smacks	Kellogg's	366	104
Smarties	Rowntree Mackintosh	460	per tube 205
Smash	Cadbury's	330	94
Smoked cod in butter sauce	Birds Eye		per pack 195
Smoked Dutch sausage	Sainsbury	370	105
Smoked garlic sausage	BHS	345	98
Smoked haddock, etc, *see Haddock, etc*			
Smoked haddock pie	St Michael	92	26
Smoked ham	BHS	157	44
Smoked ham pâté	Princes	325	92
Smoked ham sausage	Sainsbury	229	65
Smoked salmon, Canadian or Scotch	BHS	180	51

Product	Brand	Calories per 100g/ 100ml	Calories per oz/ pack/ portion
Smokey bacon spread	Princes	235	67
Snack crackers	Sainsbury		each 23
	Tesco	532	151
Snack Toast	Meadow Farm	414	9g serving 38, 200g pack 828
Snax	Sainsbury		per biscuit 17
Snow Caps	St Michael	343	97
Snow balls/snowballs	BHS	411	113g pack 464
	Cadbury's	499	141
	Huntley & Palmers	421	each 131
	Sainsbury		each 115
	St Michael	413	each 103
	Tunnock's		each 114
Soda bread		*264*	*75*
Soda water	Club	negl.	
	Hunts	negl.	
	Idris	negl.	
	Safeway	20–30	6–9
	Schweppes	negl.	
	Waitrose	24	7
Soft brown sugar dark	Tesco	383	109
	Waitrose	395	112
light	Tesco	289	82
	Waitrose	395	112
light golden	Whitworths	389	110
rich	Whitworths	383	109
Soft centred fruit flavours	Barker & Dobson	320	91

254

product	Brand	Calories per 100g/ 100ml	Calories per oz/ pack/ portion
soft cheese	Safeway	318	90
full fat:	Waitrose		
and chives		335	95
and onion		335	95
and pineapple		388	110
low fat	Safeway	96	27
Somerset:	Eden Vale		
high fat		321	91
low fat		135	38
medium fat/ cucumber		196	56
medium fat/onion and gherkin		201	57
medium fat/ pineapple		206	58
with garlic and herbs	St Michael	358	101
soft mints	Callard & Bowser, Nuttall	370	per sweet 15
	St Michael	365	103
soft nougat	BHS	390	70g pack 273
soufflé, chocolate	St Ivel	185	52
fruit	St Ivel	160	45
soup mixture (as sold)	Whitworths	331	94
soup see Chicken, etc			
southern Fried chicken portions	Ross	240	68
southern Fried Coat & Cook	Homepride	430	43g pack 185
soya bean oil	Alfonal	900	255

255

Product	Brand	Calories per 100g/ 100ml	Calories per oz/ pack/ portion
Soya bean pâté	Granose	132	37
Soyal beans in brine	Granose	171	48
in tomato sauce	Granose	119	34
Soya flour	Prewetts	433	123
Soya milk, liquid	Granose	51	14
Soya mince with onion (as sold)	Beanfeast	334	per pack 384
Soyapro slices,	Granose		
beef flavour		208	59
chicken flavour		243	69
Soy-O-Life tub	Alfonal	732	208
Spaghetti, boiled		*117*	*33*
raw		*378*	*107*
Spaghetti canned	Sainsbury	53	1tbsp/1oz 15
	Waitrose	60	17
long, raw	Waitrose	367	104
raw	BHS	346	98
	Buitoni	334	95
	James Marshall	320	91
	Sainsbury	388	110
Spaghetti Bolognese	Heinz	88	25
Spaghetti hoops in tomato sauce	Heinz	67	19
	Tesco	66	19
Spaghetti in tomato sauce		*59*	*17*
Spaghetti in tomato sauce	BHS	67	19
	Heinz	67	19
	Safeway	56	16
	Tesco	80	23

Product	Brand	Calories per 100g/ 100ml	Calories per oz/ pack/ portion
Spaghetti rings	Safeway	65	18
	Waitrose	60	17
with tomato sauce	Crosse & Blackwell	61	17
Spaghetti sauce mix	Colman's	370	105
(as sold)	Knorr	377	107
Spangles	Mars		per pkt 144/ per sweet 13
Spanish Omelette Mate	Campbell's	69	20
Spanish salad	Eden Vale	110	31
	Sainsbury	123	1tbsp/1oz 35
Sparkles:	Wall's		
cola, lemonade or			
strawberry			each 30
orangeade			39
Sparkling drinks,	Sainsbury	38	11½fl.oz can
ready to drink			130
Sparkling fruits/mints	Tesco	370	105
Special Cellar cider	H.P. Bulmer	56	16
Special K		*388*	*110*
Special K	Kellogg's	358	101
Special mix	Ross	55	16
Special Reserve cider			
dry	H.P. Bulmer	47	13
medium sweet	H.P. Bulmer	57	16
Special Vat cider			
(bottled or canned)	Taunton	39	1 pint 230
Speckled eggs and snowballs	Cadbury's	499	141

Product	Brand	Calories per 100g/ 100ml	Calories per oz/ pack/ portion
Spiced fruit buns	St Michael	285	81
Spiced raisin cake	St Michael	348	99
Spicy apple & sultana Viennese	Tiffany's Upper Crust	230	¼ dessert 355
Spicy apple roly	Tiffany's	260	¼ dessert 240
Spicy curry Pot Noodle	Golden Wonder		carton made up 381
Spicy sauce	O.K. (Colman's)	95	27
Spicy tomato Pot Rice	Golden Wonder		carton made up 251
Spicy vegetable spread	Waistline	85	24
Spinach, boiled		*30*	*8.5*
Spinach			
cut leaf	Birds Eye	18	5
leaf	Ross	30	8.5
fresh, frozen or canned and drained	Sainsbury	18	1tbsp/1oz 5
Spirits (70% proof)		*222*	*63*
Spirits	Sainsbury		⅙ gill 50
Splicer	Rowntree Mackintosh	420	per pack 180
Split peas see Peas			
Split tin crusty bread	St Michael	250	71
Sponge, strawberry jam	Sainsbury	364	⅕ cake/1½ oz 155
Sponge Bar	Waitrose	472	134
Sponge cake, jam filled		*302*	*86*
with fat		*464*	*132*
without fat		*301*	*85*

Product	Brand	Calories per 100g/ 100ml	Calories per oz/ pack/ portion
Sponge cake, double layer	St Michael	272	77
Sponge cake mix (as sold)	Whitworths	370	6½oz pack 682
Sponge curls, blackcurrant	St Michael	342	per cake 188
chocolate	St Michael	333	per cake 200
Sponge fingers	Huntley & Palmers	389	per biscuit 21
	Sainsbury		per biscuit 18
Sponge flan	Waitrose	198	56
Sponge flan case	Tesco	323	92
Sponge gâteau, chocolate			
buttercream	St Michael	413	117
raspberry jam	St Michael	391	111
with hazelnut filling	Sainsbury	423	1/5 cake/1½ oz 180
Sponge mallows	St Michael	410	per mallow 89
Sponge pudding, steamed		*344*	*98*
Sponge round	Sainsbury	300	1/5 cake/1oz 85
Sponge sandwich	Sainsbury	376	1/7 cake/1½oz 160
	Waitrose	472	134
chocolate	St Michael	323	92
jam and vanilla	Lyons	361	per cake 892
jam buttercream	St Michael	353	100
vanilla	St Michael	322	91
with lemon/orange	Tiffany's	423	¼ cake 211

Product	Brand	Calories per 100g/ 100ml	Calories per oz/ pack/ portion
Sports biscuits	BHS	481	136
Spotted Dick	St Michael	361	102
	Tiffany's	310	¼ pudding 26⁹
Sprats, fried *(with bones)*		*441* *388*	*125* *110*
Spring greens (boiled)		*10*	*3*
Spring greens	Ross	25	7
	Sainsbury	35	1tbsp/1oz 10
Spring onions, raw		*35*	*10*
Spring vegetable soup canned	Heinz	43	12
condensed (undiluted)	Granny's Batchelors	37	10
dried (as sold)	5-Minute		per pack 88
	Tesco	234	66
dried (made up)	Chef Box Maggi	16	4.5
	Quick Cook	19	5.5
	Sainsbury	7 (100ml)	½ pint 20
Florida (dried, as sold)	Knorr	282	80
Sprouts *see* Brussels sprouts			
Square loaf	St Michael	237	67
Stackers	Cadbury's	550	156
Star Bar	Cadbury's	507	144
Star mousse	Tudor	150	43
Starship 4	Wall's		each 35
Steak (grilled)	Tesco	234	66

Product	Brand	Calories per 100g/ 100ml	Calories per oz/ pack/ portion
Steak, kidney and vegetable soup (undiluted)	Campbell's Main Course	48	14
Steak and kidney pie, individual		*323*	*92*
pastry top only		*286*	*81*
Steak and kidney pie for 1 person	Brains		per pie 1535
for 1 person	Birds Eye		per pie 370
for 2–3 people	Birds Eye		per pie 1120
large	BHS	405	per pie 1840
small	BHS	254	per pie 386
	Fray Bentos	190	54
113g/4oz	Kraft	394	per pie 445
340g/12oz	Kraft	310	per pie 1055
family	Ross	200	57
individual	Ross	300	85
	Safeway	302	87
4½oz	Sainsbury	250	per pie 320
frozen, 15oz	Sainsbury	263	per pie 1120
large, 20oz	Sainsbury	247	¼ pie 350
rich pastry	St Michael	305	86
small	St Michael	303	86
standard	St Michael	296	84
canned	Tesco	198	56
fresh	Tesco	288	82
frozen	Tesco	285	81
4½oz oval, baked	Tiffany's	255	per pie 325
5oz round, baked	Tiffany's	230	per pie 326
1lb, baked	Tiffany's	260	¼ pie 295
frozen	Waitrose	303	86
Steak and kidney pie filling	Fray Bentos	120	34

Product	Brand	Calories per 100g/ 100ml	Calories per oz/ pack/ portion
Steak and kidney pudding	BHS	102	191g pudding 195
	Fray Bentos	200	57
	Goblin	200	142g pudding 285
	Kraft	281	121g/4½oz pudding 340
	Ross	260	74
5½oz	Sainsbury	238	per pudding 370
large, 16oz	Sainsbury	238	¼ pudding 270
large	Tesco	274	78
small	Tesco	294	83
Steak and kidney stew	Campbell's	48	14
Steak and mushroom pie, 1½lb, baked	Tiffany's	240	¼ pie 430
Steak and mushroom pudding	Tesco	285	81
Steak and mushroom pie filling	Fray Bentos	115	33
Steak and onion pie, 5½oz	Sainsbury	314	per pie 490
Steak and onion pie filling	Fray Bentos	110	31
Steak and vegetable pie	BHS	241	per pie 1124
Steak pie canned, 7½oz	Sainsbury	117	per pie 250

Product	Brand	Calories per 100g/ 100ml	Calories per oz/ pack/ portion
Steak pie			
canned, 15½oz	Sainsbury	117	per pie 510
fresh, 5½oz	Sainsbury	285	per pie 445
topcrust	St Michael	203	58
with onion	St Michael	271	77
	Tesco	215	61
Steak pudding		223	63
Steak seasoning	Tesco	150	43
Steakburgers, 4oz, as sold	Tiffany's	250	per burger 280
Steakhouse grills	Birds Eye		per grill, grilled or fried 240
Steaklets	Birds Eye		per steaklet, grilled or fried 200
	Danish Prime	225	64
	Ross	340	96
Stem ginger biscuits	Prewetts	474	134
Stew pack	Sainsbury	18	1 tbsp/1oz 5
Stewed steak (canned)	Waitrose	141	40
Stewed steak and gravy (canned)		176	50
Stewed steak and gravy (canned)	Sainsbury	173	15oz can 735
	Tesco	167	47
Stewing steak			
raw, lean and fat		176	50
stewed, lean and fat		223	63
Stewpack vegetables (frozen)	Tesco	25	7

Product	Brand	Calories per 100g/ 100ml	Calories per oz/ pack/ portion
Stick, crusty	St Michael	250	71
Stilton cheese	St Ivel	375	106
	St Michael	418	119
blue	Sainsbury	370	105
	Waitrose	476	135
white	Sainsbury	335	95
	Waitrose	476	135
Stir fry vegetables (as sold)	Ross	60	17
Stock cubes *see under flavours*			
Stockpot (undiluted)	Campbell's	60	17
Stollen	St Michael	343	97
Stout, bottled		*37*	*10*
extra		*39*	*11*
Straight spaghetti	Crosse & Blackwell	57	16
Strawberries			
canned		*81*	*23*
canned	Baxters	86	10¼oz/290g can 249 15oz/425g can 366 19oz/538g can 464
	Safeway	nil	nil
canned (drained)	Tesco	78	22
canned (inc. syrup)	Hartley's	115	33
	Sainsbury	75	1 tbsp/1oz 21
fresh		*26*	*7.5*
fresh or frozen	Sainsbury	26	7.5
frozen	Waitrose	25	7

264

Product	Brand	Calories per 100g/ 100ml	Calories per oz/ pack/ portion
Strawberry and cream mousse	Tesco	161	46
	Waitrose	120	34
Strawberry and vanilla ice cream	Tudor	190	54
Strawberry bars	Palm	400	113
Strawberry blancmange mix (as sold)	Brown & Polson	328	93
Strawberry conserve	BHS	260	74
Strawberry cream filled bar	St Michael	420	119
Strawberry delight (made up)	St Michael	116	33
	Tesco	134	38
Strawberry dessert	Waitrose	465	132
Strawberry dessert sauce	HP Foods	170	48
	Lyons Maid	264	75
	Tesco	315	89
	Wall's	112	250g pack 280
Strawberry dessert topping	Colman's	280	79
Strawberry drink	Cresta	33	9.5
Strawberry flake	Sainsbury		per cake 175
Strawberry flan filling	Armour	130	37
Strawberry flavour cordial (undiluted)	Quosh	118	33
Strawberry flavoured milk drink	St Michael	75	21
Strawberry gâteau	Birds Eye		1/6 cake 280
Strawberry ice cream	Sainsbury	176	1oz/2fl.oz 50
	Tudor	170	65

Product	Brand	Calories per 100g/ 100ml	Calories per oz/ pack/ portion
Strawberry ice cream			
individual slice	Wall's		per slice 60
soft serve	Tudor	180	51
Strawberry jam	Chivers		
	Extra	225	64
	Hartley's	255	72
	Moorhouse	255	72
	Robertson's	251	71
	Safeway	255	72
	Tesco	279	79
	Tesco Extra	268	76
	Waitrose	261	74
Strawberry jam sponge	Sainsbury	364	1/5 cake/ 1½oz 155
Strawberry jelly (as sold)	Chivers	285	81
	Waitrose	258	73
Strawberry Jelly Cream	Chivers	370	105
Strawberry marshmallow sundae	Wall's	174	321g pack 560
Soft Scoop	Wall's		2 litre pack 2040
Strawberry meringue	St Michael	321	91
Strawberry Mivvi	Lyons Maid		each 78
Strawberry mousse	Birds Eye		per tub 110
	Tesco	161	46
	Waitrose	95	27
Strawberry Munch Bunch	Eden Vale	105	30

Product	Brand	Calories per 100g/ 100ml	Calories per oz/ pack/ portion
Strawberry pie filling	Sainsbury	123	1 tbsp/2oz 70
	Tesco	84	24
Strawberry preserve Today's Recipe	Baxters	260	340g jar 884
	Robertson's	180	51
Strawberry ripple, Easy Scoop	Tesco	169	48
Strawberry ripple slice	Wall's		273g pack 495
Strawberry roll	St Michael	350	99
	Tesco	374	106
Strawberry split	Wall's		each 80
Strawberry sponge pudding	Heinz	285	81
Strawberry sundae	BHS	188	75g pack 141
	Eden Vale	119	34
Strawberry Sundae Best	St Ivel	185	52
Strawberry supermousse	Birds Eye		per tub 120
Strawberry supreme dessert	Sainsbury		pkt made up 445
Strawberry Two Shakes	Kellogg's	360 (dry)	½ sachet (20g) + milk 273
Strawberry vanilla Swiss roll	Waitrose	360	102
Strawberry whip	St Michael	151	43
Strawberry yogurt/ yoghurt	BHS	80	per pack 120
	St Michael	93	26
	Ski	91	26
	Waitrose	95	27

Product	Brand	Calories per 100g/ 100ml	Calories per oz/ pack/ portion
Strawberry/chocolate Twin Pack Soft Scoop ice cream	Wall's		2 litre pack 1930
Strawberry/vanilla Twin Pack Soft Scoop ice cream	Wall's		2 litre pack 1845
Strike Cola	Barr	32	9
Strong ale		*72*	*20*
Strong ale	Sainsbury	69	½ pint 195
Strongbow cider			
bottled	H.P. Bulmer	36	10
draught	H.P. Bulmer	35	10
Stuffed Manzanilla olives	Crosse & Blackwell	45	13
Suet, block		*895*	*254*
shredded		*826*	*234*
Suet	Safeway	925	262
	Tesco	826	234
	Waitrose	924	262
Suet pudding, steamed		*333*	*94*
SUGAR			
all types	Sainsbury	370	1 tbsp/1oz 105
brown crystal	Tesco	394	112
candy	Tesco	394	112
demerara		*394*	*112*
demerara	Safeway	394	112
	Tesco	394	112
	Waitrose	395	112
	Whitworths	394	112

Product	Brand	Calories per 100g/ 100ml	Calories per oz/ pack/ portion
SUGAR			
natural raw cane	Tesco	394	112
Muscovado	Tesco	383	109
rainbow crystal	Tesco	394	112
soft dark brown	Tesco	383	109
	Waitrose	395	112
soft light brown	Tesco	289	82
	Waitrose	395	112
soft light golden brown	Whitworths	389	110
soft rich brown	Whitworths	383	109
white		*394*	*112*
Sugar Puffs		348	99
Sugar Puffs	Quaker Oats	368	104
Sugar strands, assorted	Tesco	370	105
chocolate	Tesco	418	119
Sultana and Bramley apple cake	St Michael	283	80
Sultana Bran	Kellogg's	310	88
Sultana cake	Waitrose	332	94
Sultana cookies	St Michael	452	per biscuit 75
	Waitrose	480	136
Sultana cut cake	St Michael	342	97
Sultana fruit cake (580g)	BHS	371	105
Sultana Devon scones	St Michael	308	87
Sultanas, dried		*250*	*71*
Sultanas, dried	Sainsbury	247	1 tbsp/1oz 70
	Tesco	250	71

269

Product	Brand	Calories per 100g/100ml	Calories per oz/pack/portion
Sultanas, dried	Waitrose	250	71
	Whitworths	250	71
Suncrush drinks *see Lemon, etc*			
Sundae Best			
peach	St Ivel	180	51
strawberry	St Ivel	185	52
Sunflower oil	BHS	899	255
	Safeway	900	255
	St Michael	899	255
	Tesco	932	264
	Waitrose	924	262
Sunflower seed oil	Alfonal	900	255
Sunfruit drink	St Michael	47	13
Sunny sauce	O.K.		
	Colman's	85	24
Sunnybisk	Granose	360	102
Sun-O-Life block or tub	Alfonal	732	208
Sun-O-Life oil	Alfonal	900	255
Sun-Pat products *see Peanut butter, etc*			
Super Noodles (made up)	Kellogg's	136	39
Super toffee (bag)	Sharps		per pack 377 per sweet 28
Superstar mousse	Tudor	160	45
Superwhip	Birds Eye		per tub 885
Supreme (as sold)	Beanfeast	295	per pack 339
Supreme chicken soup	Sainsbury	74	½ pint 210
Supreme consommé	Sainsbury	21	½ pint 60

Product	Brand	Calories per 100g/ 100ml	Calories per oz/ pack/ portion
Supreme dessert:	Sainsbury		
banana			pkt made up 450
butterscotch			pkt made up 480
chocolate			pkt made up 485
strawberry			pkt made up 445
Sutherlands pastes	Quaker Oats	185	52
Swede, diced	Ross	20	6
Swedes, boiled		*18*	*5*
raw		*21*	*6*
Swedes	Sainsbury	18	5
Sweet and sour chicken	Birds Eye Snackpot		per pack 220 per pot 251
Sweet and sour Cook-in-Sauce	Homepride	51	376g pack 190
Sweet and sour Cooking-In sauce	Baxters	89	425g can 377
Sweet and sour pork	Birds Eye		per pack, fried 530
Sweet and sour Pot Noodle	Golden Wonder		carton made up 347
Sweet and sour Pour Over sauce	Crosse & Blackwell	112	32
Sweet and sour sauce mix (as sold)	Colman's Knorr	320 381	91 108
Sweet mango chutney	Crosse & Blackwell	229	65

Product	Brand	Calories per 100g/ 100ml	Calories per oz/ pack/ portion
Sweet mixed pickles	Crosse & Blackwell	131	37
Sweet piccalilli	Epicure	77	22
	Haywards	75	22
Sweet pickle	BHS	85	24
	Epicure	134	38
	Happy Farm	134	38
	Tesco	172	49
Sweet potatoes, boiled		85	24
raw		91	26
Sweetbread, lamb, fried		230	65
raw		131	37
Sweetcorn *see also Corn, Corn on the Cob*			
Sweetcorn			
canned drained	Tesco	106	30
canned kernels		76	22
fresh, frozen, or			
canned and drained	Sainsbury	88	1 tbsp/1oz 25
frozen	Birds Eye	106	30
	Ross	110	31
Sweetcorn and peppers, canned drained	Tesco	109	31
Sweetex liquid	Crookes	521	40ml pack 208
powder	Crookes	360	325g pack 1170
tablets	Crookes	nil	
Sweetmeal,			
milk chocolate	BHS	505	143
	Tesco	504	143
plain chocolate	BHS	500	142
	Tesco	499	141

Product	Brand	Calories per 100g/ 100ml	Calories per oz/ pack/ portion
Swiss chocolate:	St Michael		
milk		533	151
plain		524	149
soft filled milk		614	174
Swiss creams	Tesco	498	141
Swiss Gruyère spread	Tesco	395	112
Swiss Knight cheese:	Nestlé		
assorted variety pack		321	91
assorted variety pack (spreads)		283	80
medium fat processed		321	91
slices (cheese spread)		306	87
Swiss rolls *see Jam, etc; also Junior*			
Swiss style cereal	Safeway	394	112
	Sainsbury	353	1 tbsp/½oz 50
	Tesco	374	106
Syllabub	Eden Vale	281	80
Syrup, golden		*298*	*84*
Syrup, golden	Sainsbury	317	1 tbsp/1oz 90
	Tesco	303	86
Syrup pudding (foil basin)	Sainsbury		whole 715
Syrup sponge, golden (canned)	Sainsbury	275	10½oz can 820
Syrup sponge pudding, all butter	St Michael	366	104

Product	Brand	Calories per 100g/ 100ml	Calories per oz/ pack/ portion
Tab	Coca Cola		325ml negl.
Table Water:	Carr's		
large			per biscuit 31
small			per biscuit 14
Tagliatelle/tagliatelle verdi (as sold)	Buitoni	334	95
Tandoori chicken	St Michael	240	68
Tandoori Marinade curry mix (as sold)	Colman's	215	61
Tangerine jelly dessert (as sold)	Chivers	290	82
	Waitrose	258	73
Tangerine marmalade	Rose's	260	74
Tangerines		*34*	*9.5*
(with peel and pips)		*23*	*6.5*
Tangerines	Sainsbury	24	1×3oz 20
Tango drinks *see Lemon, etc*			
Tangy Lemon Shred	Chivers	260	74
Orange Shred	Chivers	260	74
Tapioca (raw)		*359*	*102*
Tapioca (both types), raw	Safeway	359	102
(medium or seed pearl), raw	Whitworths	359	102
Tapioca pudding canned	Sainsbury	106	15½oz can 465
creamed, canned	Ambrosia	89	25
	Safeway	144	45
	Waitrose	130	37
Tarragon and Thyme mustard	Colman's	125	35

Product	Brand	Calories per 100g/100ml	Calories per pack/portion
Tartare sauce	Colman's	255	72
	Safeway	310	88
	Sainsbury	229	1 tbsp/1oz 65
	St Michael	247	70
	Tesco	277	79
	Waistline	151	43
Tastex	Granose	208	59
Taunton draught cider, dry	Taunton	29	1 pint 170
Taxi	Macdonalds		per biscuit 82
Tea, infusion		negl.	
Tea Biscuits finger	Pennywise		per biscuit 23
milk chocolate topped	St Michael	474	per biscuit 72
Tea cakes	St Michael	260	74
milk chocolate	Tesco	427	121
Tea finger biscuits	Sainsbury		per biscuit 25
	Waitrose	448	127
Teacakes	Tunnock's		per biscuit 89
Teatime Batch	St Michael	249	71
Teatime Dainties	Sainsbury		per cake 90
Tender Bits	Granose	79	22
Texan	Rowntree	430	per pack 180
Thick soups, etc, see *Chicken*, etc			
Thin arrowroot biscuits	Crawford		per biscuit 32
Thin wheat biscuits	Sainsbury		per biscuit 25
Thousand Island dressing	Kraft	392	111

Product	Brand	Calories per 100g/ 100ml	Calories per oz/ pack/ portion
Three Fruits marmalade	Baxters	253	12oz/340g jar 860
Thyme, rubbed	Tesco	250	71
Ticket	Cadbury's	511	145
Tiffany wafers, chocolate	Peek Frean	444	per biscuit 69
lemon or orange	Peek Frean	425	per biscuit 66
Tiger sauce	Fletchers	96	27
Tigertots	Rowntree Mackintosh	380	108
Tip Top	Nestlé	110	31
Tit Bits sauce	Fletchers	96	27
Tizer	Barr	40	11
Toast Toppers *see under flavours*			
Toasted bran	Meadow Farm	350	28.3g serving 100
Toasted bread		297	84
Toasted farmhouse bran	Weetabix	300	30g serving 90 + ½ cup/5fl.oz milk 81 = 171
Toasting loaf, small	St Michael	269	76
Toffee almond ice cream	St Michael	225	64
Toffee assortment	Parkinsons	416	117
	Tesco	480	136
Toffee Brazils	Tesco	420	119
Toffee Crisp	Rowntree Mackintosh	510	per pack 195
Toffee Crumble	Lyons Maid		each 180

Product	Brand	Calories per 100g/ 100ml	Calories per oz/ pack/ portion
Toffee crunch sundae Soft Scoop	Wall's	181	2 litre/324g pack 588
Toffee Fudge – Caramella Italiano	Wall's	206	1 litre/545g pack 1125
Toffee ripple family brick	Lyons Maid		per pack 429
Toffees, Double Devon	St Michael	440	125
Toffees, mixed		*430*	*122*
Toffo	Rowntree Mackintosh	455	per pack 235
Tom & Jerry bars chews or stickpacks	Wall's	381	each 50 108
Tomato, bacon and ham Omelette Mate	Campbell's	103	29
Tomato, cheese and onion pizza (6 per pack)	St Michael	203	58
Tomato and apple chutney	Happy Farm	170	48
Tomato and bacon soup (as sold)	Knorr Quick Soups	373	106
Tomato and beef soup (as sold)	Knorr Hearty Soups	335	95
	Knorr Quick Soups	355	101
Tomato and cheese party pizzas (4 per pack)	BHS	315	per pack 1040

Product	Brand	Calories per 100g/ 100ml	Calories per oz/ pack/ portion
Tomato and cheese pizza			
93g	Birds Eye	290	per pizza 270
227g	Birds Eye	277	per pizza 630
5in	Ross	240	68
wholemeal, 5in	Ross	240	68
Tomato and chilli	BHS	109	31
relish	Tesco	109	31
Tomato and ham Pasta Menu	Crosse & Blackwell	86	24
Tomato and ham Pour Over sauce	Crosse & Blackwell	94	27
Tomato and mushroom spaghetti sauce	Campbell's	73	21
Tomato and onion Cook-in-Sauce	Homepride	69	376g pack 26
Tomato and vegetable juice	Campbell's	20	6
Tomato and vegetable soup	Chef Chunky	52	15
Italian	5-Minute		per pack 148
with croûtons	Cup-a-Soup Special	333	per portion 110
Tomato chutney		*154*	*44*
Tomato chutney	Crosse & Blackwell	144	41
Tomato cocktail	Club	26	113ml 30
Tomato juice (canned)		*16*	*4.5*
Tomato juice	Britvic	26	7
	Club	26	113ml 30
	Heinz	24	7

278

Product	Brand	Calories per 100g/ 100ml	Calories per oz/ pack/ portion
Tomato juice	Libby	20	6
	Sainsbury	21	¼ pint 30
	Tesco	21	6
	Waitrose	14	4
Tomato juice cocktail	Britvic	26	7
	Hunts	16	4.5
	Schweppes	17	5
Tomato ketchup		98	28
Tomato ketchup	Chef	109	31
	Daddies	105	30
	HP Foods	100	28
	Heinz	108	31
	Libby	106	30
	Tesco	100	28
	Waistline	50	14
Tomato paste	Napolina	112	32
Tomato pickle	Baxters	188	291g jar 427
Tomato puffs	BHS	550	156
Tomato purée		67	19
Tomato purée	Buitoni	72	20
	Tesco	71	20
Tomato relish	BHS	109	31
	Tesco	93	26
Tomato rice soup	Campbell's	93	26 undiluted
Tomato sauce		86	24
Tomato sauce	Daddies	66	19
	Sainsbury	123	1tbsp/1oz 35
Tomato soup *see also Cream of tomato*			
Tomato soup canned	BHS	74	per can 315
	Granny's	43	12

Product	Brand	Calories per 100g/ 100ml	Calories per oz/ pack/ portion
Tomato soup			
canned	Sainsbury	56	½ pint 160
condensed	Campbell's		
(undiluted)	Harvest	66	19
	Campbell's		
	Condensed	68	19
dried (as sold)	Cup-a-Soup	361	per portion 83
	Knorr		
	Quick	386	20.5g pkt 79
	Tesco	348	99
dried (made up)	Chef Box	36	10
	Maggi		
	Quick Cook	38	11
low calorie	Heinz	24	7
	Waistline	22	6
traditional	5-Minute		per pack 267
Tomato soup with	Frank		
prawns	Cooper	41	15oz can 180
Tomato spaghetti sauce	Campbell's	90	26
Tomatoes, canned		*12*	*3.5*
Tomatoes			
canned	Armour	12	3.5
	BHS	17	14oz can 70
	Napolina	21	6
	Waitrose	21	6
canned drained	Tesco	21	6
fresh or canned			
and drained	Sainsbury	14	4
fried		*69*	*20*
raw		*14*	*4*

Product	Brand	Calories per 100g/ 100ml	Calories per oz/ pack/ portion
Tome au raisin cheese	Sainsbury	265	75
Tongue			
canned		*213*	*60*
cooked	Sainsbury	282	1 thin slice/ 2oz 160
lamb, raw		*193*	*55*
ox, pickled, raw		*220*	*62*
boiled		*293*	*83*
sheep, stewed		*289*	*82*
Tongue sausage	BHS	254	72
Tonic water *see also Indian tonic water*			
Tonic water	Safeway	20–30	6–9
	Sainsbury	18	125ml/¼ pint 25
	Schweppes	20	6
	Waitrose	28	8
low calorie	Sainsbury	1.5	125ml/¼pint 2
slimline	Schweppes	5	1.5
Tooty Frooties	Rowntree Mackintosh	412	per bag 200
Tooty Minties	Rowntree Mackintosh	425	per bag 210
Top Cream toffee (bag)	Sharps		per pack 380 per sweet 36
Top Deck drinks *see Lemonade shandy, etc*			
Top 'n' Fill (all flavours)	Homepride	432	220g pack 950
Topic, single	Mars		per pack 246
Topside *see Beef*			

281

Product	Brand	Calories per 100g/ 100ml	Calories per oz/ pack/ portion
Tortellini	Crosse & Blackwell	106	30
Treacle, black		*257*	*73*
Treacle brittle	Callard & Bowser, Nuttall	390	per sweet 33
Treacle Crunch biscuits	Peek Frean	435	per biscuit 29
Treacle sponge pudding	Heinz	285	81
Treacle tart		*371*	*105*
Treacle tart, large	Sainsbury	370	1/6 tart/2oz 210
small	Sainsbury		per tart 140
Treacle toffee	Barker & Dobson	430	122
Treacle toffees	Callard & Bowser, Nuttall	450	per sweet 38
Trebor mints	Trebor		per pack 100 per sweet 6.5
Treets, peanut	Mars		standard pack 248 per sweet 10.5
toffee	Mars		standard pack 250 per sweet 14
Trifle		*160*	*45*
Trifle	Birds Eye		per tub 120
(average)	St Ivel	144	41
fresh cream	Sainsbury		small tub 230

282

Product	Brand	Calories per 100g/ 100ml	Calories per oz/ pack/ portion
Trifle, fresh cream	Tesco	176	50
fruit, individual	St Michael	158	45
fruit, large	St Michael	165	47
Trifle sponges	Lyons	325	per pack 631
	Sainsbury		per sponge 90
	Waitrose	198	56
Trio	Jacobs	526	per biscuit 132
Tripe, dressed		*60*	*17*
stewed		*100*	*28*
Triple Decker	Lyons	325	per cake 631
Tropical lemon drink, sparkling (canned)	Hunts	34	9.5
Trout, brown, steamed		*135*	*38*
(with bones)		*89*	*25*
Truffle bar	St Michael	500	142
TUC biscuits	Crawford		per biscuit 26
Tuna, canned	Waitrose	187	53
drained	Tesco	283	80
in brine (chunks or steak), drained	John West	110	31
in oil		*289*	*82*
in oil	Armour	289	82
	Sainsbury	247	70
in oil (chunks or steak), drained	John West	197	56
Tuna and mushroom pie, 1½lb (baked)	Tiffany's	235	¼ pie 425
Tuna fish salad	BHS	456	129

Product	Brand	Calories per 100g/ 100ml	Calories per oz/ pack/ portion
Tunes	Mars		per pack 144 per sweet 13
TURKEY	British Poultry Federation	198	56
boneless roast	St Michael	145	41
breast fillets	St Michael	115	33
breast joint with chestnut stuffing	St Michael	232	66
breast joint with pork fat	St Michael	201	57
escalopes in breadcrumbs	St Michael	212	60
kebabs	St Michael	88	25
loaf with bacon	St Michael	164	46
medallions	St Michael	204	58
raw, dark meat		*114*	*32*
raw, light meat		*103*	*29*
raw, meat and skin		*145*	*41*
raw, meat only		*107*	*30*
roast, dark meat		*148*	*42*
roast, light meat		*132*	*37*
roast, meat and skin		*171*	*48*
roast, meat only		*140*	*40*
sliced roast	St Michael	195	55
whole fresh	St Michael	157	45
Turkey, canned cured	St Michael	150	43
Turkey and bacon loaf	St Michael	259	73
Turkey and ham pie	St Michael	295	84
Turkey and ham Toast Topper	Heinz	108	31

Product	Brand	Calories per 100g/ 100ml	Calories per oz/ pack/ portion
Turkey and vegetable broth (undiluted)	Campbell's	77	22
Turkey in rich pastry	St Michael	318	90
Turkey pâté	Princes	310	88
Turkey pie (464g)	BHS		per pie 1256
Turkey savoury (as sold)	Tiffany's		per savoury 190
Turkey soup	Frank Cooper	49	15oz can 210
Turkish Delight	BHS	244	64
	Cadbury's	391	111
	Fry's	361	102
Turnip, diced	Ross	20	6
Turnips			
boiled		*14*	*4*
raw		*20*	*6*
tops, boiled		*11*	*3*
Turnips	Sainsbury	18	5
Tutti Frutti – Classico Italiano	Wall's	185	580g/1 litre pack 1075
Soft Scoop	Wall's	106	2 litre pack 2115
TVP, beef flavoured	Granose	250	71
chicken flavoured	Granose	227	64
sweet and sour flavoured	Granose	250	71
Twiglets	Sainsbury		per biscuit 3
large	Peek Frean	413	per biscuit 6
small	Peek Frean	410	per biscuit 2.5

Product	Brand	Calories per 100g/ 100ml	Calories per oz/ pack/ portion
Twigsticks	BHS	410	60
Twin lolly (multipack)	Lyons Maid		each 37
Twix, single	Mars		per pack 137
T-break	Mars		per pack 80
2-Minute Noodles:	Crosse &		
beef flavour	Blackwell	127	36
chicken flavour		124	35
Two Shakes:	Kellogg's	dry:	½ sachet (20g) +½ pint milk:
banana		360	273
chocolate		366	274
raspberry		359	273
strawberry		360	273

Product	Brand	Calories per 100g/ 100ml	Calories per oz/ pack/ portion
United biscuits	McVitie's		each 110
Valueburgers (1¾oz, as sold)	Tiffany's	255	per burger 127
Vanilla bar	Lyons Maid		each 72
Vanilla blancmange mix (as sold)	Brown & Polson	326	31g pack 101
Vanilla choc ice	Tudor	290	82
Vanilla chock stick (multipack)	Lyons Maid		each 136
Vanilla ice cream	Safeway	194	55
	Sainsbury	176	1oz/2fl. oz 50
	St Michael	172	49
	Tesco	212	60
	Tudor	170	48
cutting brick	Lyons Maid		per pack 846
Easy Scoop	Tesco	169	48
family brick	Lyons Maid		per pack 402
handy pack	Lyons Maid		per pack 261
individual slice	Wall's		each 65
Soft Service	Tudor	180	51
Vanilla Jelly Cream	Chivers	370	105
Vanilla Kup	Lyons Maid		each 84
Vanilla sponge mix (fully made up)	Sainsbury	423	1/6 cake/2½oz 300
Vanilla yogurt	Eden Vale	92	26
Veal			
cutlet, fried		*215*	*61*
fillet, raw		*109*	*31*
fillet, roast		*230*	*65*
jellied, canned		*125*	*35*

Product	Brand	Calories per 100g/ 100ml	Calories per oz/ pack/ portion
Veal Cordon Bleu (as sold)	Tiffany's	240	per pack 345
Veal portions in breadcrumbs	Sainsbury	212	3oz portion 180
Vegetable and beef soup	Batchelors		
dried (as sold)	Cup-a-soup	395	per portion 85
	Knorr Hearty	355	101
low calorie thick (dried, made up)	Heinz	23	6.5
	Sainsbury	21	½ pint 60
traditional	Batchelors 5-Minute		per pack 164
Vegetable and chicken soup (as sold)	Knorr Hearty Soups	378	107
Vegetable and lentil soup	Heinz Big Soups	48	14
Vegetable and steak pie	Fray Bentos	165	47
Vegetable broth with beef (undiluted)	Granny's	40	11
Vegetable oil		*899*	*255*
Vegetable oil	Safeway	900	255
	Tesco	932	264
	Waitrose	924	262
solidified	Armour	930	264
	BHS	900	255
Vegetable pâté	Granose	296	84
Vegetable salad	Eden Vale	141	40

Product	Brand	Calories per 100g/ 100ml	Calories per oz/ pack/ portion
Vegetable salad	Heinz	145	41
	Sainsbury	141	1 tbsp/1oz 40
	St Michael	265	75
canned	Tesco	152	43
fresh	Tesco	140	40
Vegetable soup see also Country, Cream of, Spring, etc			
Vegetable soup, canned		37	10
Vegetable soup canned	Crosse & Blackwell	48	14
	Heinz Big Soups	54	15
	Heinz Ready to Serve	53	15
	Sainsbury	28	½ pint 80
	Tesco	36	10
	Waitrose	47	14
condensed (undiluted)	Campbell's Bumper Harvest	43	12
	Campbell's Condensed	69	20
	Campbell's Main-Course	43	12
	Granny's	44	12
dried Crofters' thick	Chef Chunky	53	15
(dried, as sold)	Knorr	341	97

Product	Brand	Calories per 100g/ 100ml	Calories per oz/ pack/ portion
Vegetable soup			
farmhouse thick	Crosse & Blackwell	53	15
	Heinz	47	13
low calorie	Heinz	22	6
	Waistline	22	6
Scotch	Baxters	26	15oz/425g can 112
thick (dried, made up)	Sainsbury	21	½ pint 60
Vegetable soup with beef			
canned	Sainsbury	35	½ pint 100
dried (made up)	Chef Box	26	7.5
Vegetable soup with beef and noodles (dried, made up)	Maggi Quick Cook	24	7
Vegetable soup with lentils, Scottish	Baxters	59	17
Venison, roast		*198*	*56*
Venison soup	Frank Cooper	46	15oz can 195
Vermicelli (as sold)	Buitoni	334	95
Vermouth, dry		*118*	*33*
Vermouth, dry	Sainsbury		⅓ gill 60
Vermouth, sweet		*151*	*43*
Vermouth, sweet	Sainsbury		⅓ gill 70
Vesta meals *see under flavours*			
Vichyssoise	Baxters	45	15oz/425g can 191

Product	Brand	Calories per 100g/ 100ml	Calories per oz/ pack/ portion
Vichyssoise	Frank Cooper	39	15oz can 165
	Crosse & Blackwell	47	13
Viennese cakes, all butter (5 per pack)	St Michael	534	per cake 283
Viennese fancies	Sainsbury		per cake 130
Vimto	Barr	25	7
Vinaigrette	Eden Vale	33	9.5
low calorie	Kraft	93	tbsp (15ml) 14
Vindaloo Classic Curry	Homepride	128	383g pack 490
Vindaloo curry mix (as sold)	Colman's	335	95
Vinegar		4	1
Vinegar and oil dressing,	Tesco	152	43
low calorie	Safeway	165	47
	Waistline	170	48
Vintage marmalade	Baxters	253	12oz/340g jar 860
	Frank Cooper	263	75
Virginia sweetcorn soup (as sold)	Knorr	364	103
Vita Weat/		401	
Vita Weat Rye	Jacobs	395	per biscuit 28
Vitbe bread	St Michael	240	68
Vol au Vent cases	Birds Eye		per case 70

Product	Brand	Calories per 100g/ 100ml	Calories per oz/ pack/ portion
Wafer creams	Tunnock's		per biscuit 109
Wafer Delights	Huntley & Palmers	379	per biscuit 97
Wafer sandwich biscuits, chocolate filling	Waitrose	504	143
Wafer snack	Cadbury's	545	155
Wafers	Pennywise		per biscuit 46
Wafers, filled ice cream	Wall's	535	152 per wafer 6
Waffle wafers (lemon or orange	Meadow Farm	535	150g pack 802, 7g serving 38
Waffles	BHS	271	per waffle 70
	Ross	194	55
	St Michael	276	78
Waldorf salad	St Ivel	135	38
	St Michael	298	84
	Tesco	135	38
Walnut biscuits	Allinson	520	148
Walnut cheese	St Michael	315	89
Walnut layer cake	BHS	376	107
	Waitrose	427	121
Walnut muesli yogurt	Country Prize	88	25
Walnut sandwich cake all butter	St Michael	404	115
with buttercream	Tiffany's	428	¼ cake 267
Walnut whip, milk choc. coffee or vanilla	Rowntree	480	per whip 160
plain choc. vanilla	Mackintosh	470	per whip 155

Product	Brand	Calories per 100g/ 100ml	Calories per oz/ pack/ portion
Walnuts		525	149
(with shells)		336	95
Walnuts	Sainsbury	529	150
halves or shelled	Whitworths	525	149
pickled	Epicure	69	20
	Haywards	80	23
roasted shelled	Tesco	525	149
Warm Start	Quaker Oats	400	113
Water biscuits		440	125
Water biscuits	Jacobs	393	per biscuit 31
high baked	Tesco	394	112
Watercress, raw		14	4
Watermelon, raw		21	6
(with skin)		11	3
Weetabix		340	96
Weetabix	Weetabix	335	2 biscuits 117 +4oz milk 74 +½oz sugar 56 = 247
Weetaflakes	Weetabix	335	1oz flakes 100 +4oz milk 74 +½oz sugar 56 = 230
Weight Watchers			
cutting brick	Lyons Maid		per pack 527
family brick	Lyons Maid		per pack 251
Weiners	Granose	210	59
Welsh rarebit		365	103
Wensleydale cheese	Sainsbury	388	110
	St Michael	375	106

Product	Brand	Calories per 100g/ 100ml	Calories per oz/ pack/ portion
Wensleydale cheese	Tesco	395	112
	Waitrose	405	115
West Country draught cider:	H.P. Bulmer		
dry		35	10
extra dry		31	9
medium sweet		38	11
Wheat biscuit cereal	Waitrose	353	100
Wheat biscuits, thin	Sainsbury		per biscuit 25
Wheat bran _see Bran_			
Wheat crackers	Tesco	445	126
Wheat crispbread whole wheat with bran	Sainsbury		per piece 30
	Tesco	360	102
Wheat Crunchies	St Michael	482	137
Wheat Flakes	Force	360	102
	Sainsbury	353	4tbsp/½oz 50
Wheateats	Allinson	427	121
Wheaten crackers	St Michael	480	per cracker 29
Wheatgerm	Granose	360	102
natural	Jordans	359	102
stabilised	Allinson	345	98
Wheatmeal cake	Sainsbury	362	⅙ cake/2oz 205
Wheatmeal crisp biscuits	Sainsbury		per biscuit 20
Whelks, boiled		91	26
(with shells)		14	4
White bread		233	66
White bread	Sainsbury		thin slice 70

Product	Brand	Calories per 100g/ 100ml	Calories per oz/ pack/ portion
White bread	Sainsbury		medium slice 95 thick slice 115
sliced (medium or thin)	St Michael	228	65
White Candy products	Goodies	537	152
White pepper, ground	Whitworths	308	87
ground or whole	Tesco	275	78
White pudding		450	128
White sauce			
savoury		151	43
sweet		172	49
White sauce mix			
(as sold)	Colman's	380	108
	Knorr	354	100
(made up)	Chef Box	96	27
	Sainsbury	53	1tbsp/½oz 15
White sugar		394	112
White wine *see* Wine			
White wine Cook-in-Sauce	Homepride	78	376g pack 295
White wine Cooking-In sauce	Baxters	92	425g can 390
White wine Pour Over sauce	Crosse & Blackwell	52	15
Whitebait, fried		525	149
Whitecurrants			
raw		26	7.5
stewed with sugar		57	16
stewed without sugar		22	6

Product	Brand	Calories per 100g/ 100ml	Calories per oz/ pack/ portion
WHITING	Sainsbury	106	30
breaded (frozen)	BHS	149	42
fillets	Ross	80	23
	Waitrose	92	26
fillets or 2lb bag	St Michael	188	33
fried		*191*	*54*
fried (with bones)		*173*	*49*
smoked	Sainsbury	70	20
smoked fillets	Ross	80	23
steamed		*92*	*26*
steamed (with bones)		*63*	*18*
Whole wheat biscuit cereal	Waitrose	353	100
Whole wheat bisk cereal	Sainsbury		per biscuit 70
Wholemeal biscuits	Prewetts	516	146
Wholemeal bran biscuits	BHS	460	130
	Safeway	460	130
	St Michael	460	per biscuit 67
Wholemeal bread		*216*	*61*
Wholemeal bread	Sainsbury		thin slice 65 med. slice 85 thick slice 110
Wholenut, milk	Cadbury's	551	156
Wholewheat breakfast cereal	Tesco	336	95
Wholewheat flakes	Prewetts	359	102
Wholewheat museli	Tesco	377	107
Wild bramble jelly	Baxters	260	12oz/340g jar 884

Product	Brand	Calories per 100g/100ml	Calories per oz/pack/portion
WINE			
dry	Sainsbury	67	¼ pint glass 95
medium	Sainsbury	74	¼ pint glass 105
red		*68*	*19*
rosé, medium		*71*	*20*
sweet	Sainsbury	92	¼ pint glass 130
white, dry		*66*	*19*
white, medium		*75*	*21*
white, sparkling		*76*	*22*
white, sweet		*94*	*27*
Wine gums	Bassett's	342	97
	St Michael	342	97
mini	St Michael	342	97
Winkles, boiled (weighed with shells)		*74*	*21*
		14	*4*
Winner	Jacobs	495	per biscuit 98
Wings	Peek Frean	489	per biscuit 3
Wizard mouse, chocolate	St Ivel	175	50
fruit	St Ivel	180	51
Woodpecker cider:	H.P. Bulmer		
draught		35	10
dry (bottled)		30	8.5
medium sweet (bottled)		28	8
Woppas	Wall's		each 40
Worcestershire sauce	Lea & Perrins	72	20

Product	Brand	Calories per 100g/ 100ml	Calories per oz/ pack/ portion
Yam, boiled		119	34
raw		131	37
Yeast, bakers', compressed		53	15
dried		169	48
Yeast, dried active baking	Allinson	326	92
Yeast extract, savoury spread	Safeway	190	55
Yo Yo:	Macdonalds		
mint			per biscuit 101
orange			per biscuit 100
toffee			per biscuit 93
Yogo (all flavours)		385	109
Yogurt/Yoghurt *see also Ski*			
YOGURT/YOGHURT			
apricot	Waitrose	95	27
apricot and almond	St Michael	108	31
average	Countess	117	33
banana	Eden Vale	92	26
	Sainsbury	102	sm. tub/¼ pint 145
	Waitrose	95	27
black cherry	BHS	80	150g pack 120
	Sainsbury	123	sm. tub/¼ pint 175
	St Michael	97	27
	Waitrose	95	27
blackcurrant	Waitrose	95	27

Product	Brand	Calories per 100g/ 100ml	Calories per oz/ pack/ portion
YOGURT			
Caribbean	BHS	83	150g pack 125
champagne rhubarb	BHS	80	150g pack 121
chocolate	Eden Vale	96	27
	Sainsbury	127	tub/¼ pint 180
farmhouse			
blackcurrant	BHS	111	31
farmhouse			
gooseberry	BHS	115	33
farmhouse natural	BHS	115	33
farmhouse			
raspberry	BHS	111	31
flavoured		*81*	*23*
fruit		*95*	*27*
fruit	Safeway	62	18
grapefruit	Country		
muesli	Prize	83	24
hazelnut		*106*	*30*
hazelnut	Sainsbury	106	sm. tub/¼ pint 150
	Waitrose	95	27
Jaffa orange	St Michael	85	24
lemon	Waitrose	95	27
lemon/lime	Eden Vale	92	26
mandarin	Waitrose	95	27
muesli	Country		
	Prize	92	27
	St Michael	112	32
natural (low fat)		*52*	*15*
natural	BHS	60	150g pack 90
	Eden Vale	70	20

Product	Brand	Calories per 100g/ 100ml	Calories per oz/ pack/ portion
YOGURT, natural	St Ivel	60	17
	Waitrose	56	16
natural, unsweetened	Sainsbury	46	tub/¼ pint 65
	St Michael	69	20
natural and grapefruit	Eden Vale	86	24
natural and honey	Eden Vale	90	26
other fruit	Sainsbury	70	sm. tub/¼ pint 100
peach melba	BHS	79	150g pack 119
	St Michael	101	29
pineapple	St Michael	83	24
	Waitrose	95	27
prune	St Michael	101	29
raisin and brazil nut	Waitrose	95	27
raspberry	St Michael	101	29
	Waitrose	95	27
red cherry	Waitrose	95	27
strawberry	BHS	80	150g pack 120
	St Michael	93	26
	Waitrose	95	27
sweetened	Waitrose	88/95	25/27
vanilla	Eden Vale	92	26
Walnut muesli	Country Prize	88	25
Yogurt dressing	Heinz	285	81
Yorkie:	Rowntree Mackintosh		
milk chocolate		525	per pack 320

Product	Brand	Calories per 100g/ 100ml	Calories per oz/ pack/ portion
raisin and biscuit		470	per pack 270
peanut		545	per pack 315
Yorkshire pudding		*215*	*61*
Yorkshire pudding and pancake mix (as sold)	Whitworths	348	4½ oz pack 444
Yorkshire recipe butter mints/treacle mints	Callard & Bowser, Nuttall	390	per sweet 28
Yule log (rum)	Lyons	405	per cake 944
Zanzibar biscuits	Huntley & Palmers	419	per biscuit 56
Zest (all flavours)		386	109
Zing drinks *see Orange, etc*			
Zoom	Lyons Maid		each 44